Labor and Delivery from a Public Health Perspective

Edited by Alexander Juusela

Published in London, United Kingdom

Labor and Delivery from a Public Health Perspective
http://dx.doi.org/10.5772/intechopen.1004503
Edited by Alexander Juusela

Contributors
A. Geetha Lakshmi, Ahmedin Aliyi Usso, Alexander Juusela, Alexander Juusela, Angelline Goshomi, Anjalakshi Chandrasekar, Benjamin Joseph Nggada, Bernadether Terentius Rugumisa, Efuetnkeng Bechem, Fatemeh Ahadi Yulghunlu, Habtamu Alemu Tena, N. Bhavatharini, Omur Cinar Elci, Owen Goshomi, Pikee Saxena, Rajesh Jain, Rebecca Bradley, Sofia Beatriz Edmonson, Tesfahun Simon Hadaro, Unice Goshomi, V. Seshiah

First published in London, United Kingdom, 2025 by IntechOpen
IntechOpen is the global imprint of INTECHOPEN LIMITED, registered in England and Wales, registration number: 11086078, 167-169 Great Portland Street, London, W1W 5PF, United Kingdom

For EU product safety concerns: IN TECH d.o.o., Prolaz Marije Krucifikse Kozulić 3, 51000 Rijeka, Croatia, info@intechopen.com or visit our website at intechopen.com.

British Library Cataloguing-in-Publication Data
A catalogue record for this book is available from the British Library

Labor and Delivery from a Public Health Perspective
Edited by Alexander Juusela
p. cm.

This title is part of the Obstetrics and Gynecology Book Series, Volume 8
Topic: Maternal-fetal Medicine
Series Editor: Zouhair O. Amarin
Topic Editor: Artúr Beke

Print ISBN 978-1-83634-041-6
Online ISBN 978-1-83634-040-9
eBook (PDF) ISBN 978-1-83634-042-3
ISSN 3049-706X

If disposing of this product, please recycle the paper responsibly.

IntechOpen Book Series
Obstetrics and Gynecology
Volume 8

Aims and Scope of the Series

Obstetrics and Gynecology field typically covers several subspecialties that include maternal-fetal medicine, gynecologic oncology, reproductive endocrinology and subfertility, urogynecology and female pelvic reconstructive surgery, critical care medicine, complex family planning, pediatric and adolescent gynecology, menopausal and geriatric gynecology, and minimally invasive gynecologic surgery.
Apart from being diverse, obstetrics and gynecology is a challenging and demanding specialty. It combines medical and surgical skills.
The sequence of books in this series will have certain characteristics in common that will be recognized as part of the same informative multi-volume book programme.

Meet the Series Editor

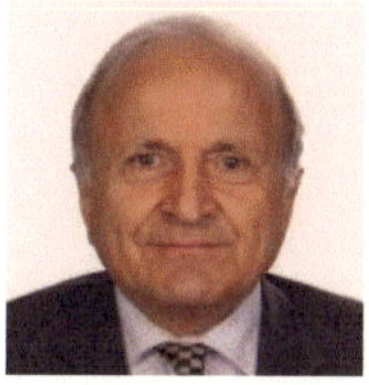

Zouhair Amarin is a Professor of Obstetrics and Gynaecology at the Jordan University of Science and Technology. He was previously a lecturer at the University of Glasgow, Scotland, a senior lecturer at the University of Nottingham, England, and the dean of the Faculty of Medicine at Mutah University, Jordan. Professor Amarin is a fellow of the Royal College of Obstetricians and Gynaecologists, and the Faculty of Public Health, London. He holds master's degrees in medical science and medical education. He is a pioneer in IVF and was the first in the world to develop microsurgical epididymis sperm aspiration for clinical use. He also discovered a surgical procedure for critical ovarian hyperstimulation syndrome. Professor Amarin has edited books, authored book chapters, and published more than 130 papers. He is the recipient of eight awards.

Meet the Volume Editor

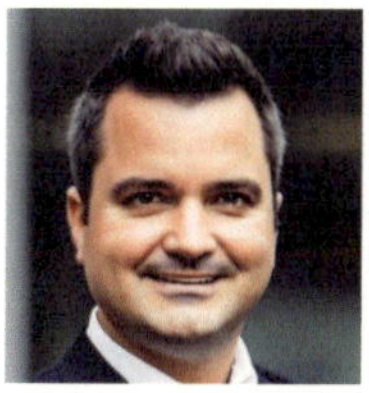

Alex Juusela, MD, MPH, FACOG, is a board-certified obstetrician-gynecologist and maternal-fetal medicine specialist. He trained at the NIH Perinatology Research Branch at Wayne State University and currently serves as MFM faculty at Newark Beth Israel Medical Center. A dedicated educator and clinician, he has earned multiple honors, including the ACOG National Faculty Award. His work spans maternal health, perinatal outcomes, and medical education, with over a dozen peer-reviewed publications, book chapters, and national committee appointments. Dr. Juusela blends clinical excellence with a passion for maternal health equity, quality improvement, and systems-based care, contributing to national initiatives that shape obstetric care, patient education, and public health policy.

Contents

Preface

Women are not dying because of diseases we cannot treat. They are dying because societies have yet to make the decision that their lives are worth saving.

Mahmoud Fahmy Fathalla (1935 – 2023)

The process of childbirth stands at the intersection of biology, culture, and medical science, reflecting both the constancy of human reproduction and the profound evolution of obstetric care over centuries. In antiquity, childbirth was an event deeply embedded in spiritual and communal frameworks, attended by birthing attendants whose knowledge was transmitted through generations. Egyptian medical papyri, Hippocratic treatises, and Roman texts reveal early understandings of obstetric techniques, though these were often interwoven with mythological interpretations and ritualistic interventions. Across civilizations, childbirth was both a sacred and perilous event, where maternal survival was uncertain, and interventions were rudimentary at best.

The medieval and early modern periods saw midwives maintaining a central role in birthing care, though their practices were often constrained by limited empirical knowledge and deeply ingrained superstitions. The early modern era heralded a shift with the increasing involvement of male physicians, catalyzing the gradual medicalization of childbirth. By the 18th and 19th centuries, the advent of forceps and other instrumental interventions marked an inflection point, enabling assisted deliveries while simultaneously introducing new risks due to inadequate antiseptic techniques. Maternal mortality remained alarmingly high, largely due to puerperal infections and the absence of standardized medical oversight.

The 20th century ushered in an unprecedented transformation in obstetric care, driven by advancements in germ theory, antibiotics, anesthesia, and surgical techniques. The institutionalization of childbirth within hospitals facilitated access to life-saving medical interventions, yet it also contributed to the increasing medicalization of labor. The routine use of cesarean sections, while invaluable in cases of obstetric emergencies, has raised concerns regarding its overuse, leading to a critical reevaluation of best practices in labor management.

From a public health perspective, the contemporary landscape of maternal care presents both remarkable progress and persistent inequities. While high-income nations have witnessed dramatic declines in maternal mortality, vast disparities remain, particularly in low-resource settings where access to skilled birth attendants and emergency obstetric care is often inadequate. Social determinants of health, ranging from economic stability to healthcare infrastructure, continue to profoundly influence maternal and neonatal outcomes. Addressing these systemic issues necessitates a comprehensive, evidence-based approach that transcends clinical settings and incorporates broader policy initiatives.

The over-medicalization of childbirth in some regions stands in contrast to the underutilization of essential obstetric interventions in others. This dichotomy underscores the need for a recalibrated approach that prioritizes the judicious use of medical interventions while reinforcing the value of physiological birth, midwifery-led care, and community-based models of maternal support. Operative vaginal delivery, for instance, remains an underutilized but crucial alternative to cesarean delivery, offering a means to reduce surgical morbidity when appropriately indicated.

Equally imperative is the need to integrate respectful maternity care into obstetric practice. Ensuring that all individuals experience childbirth in a dignified, patient-centered manner is fundamental to advancing maternal health. The elimination of obstetric violence, the promotion of intrapartum companionship, and the integration of culturally competent care models are essential in fostering trust in healthcare systems and improving health-seeking behaviors.

A robust public health framework for labor and delivery must be dynamic, responsive to emerging evidence, and adaptable to the diverse needs of populations worldwide. By harmonizing technological advancements with foundational principles of maternal care—respect, equity, and safety—societies can work toward a future in which both medical excellence and human dignity support every birth. Through interdisciplinary collaboration among clinicians, policymakers, and public health professionals, meaningful progress in maternal health can be realized, ensuring that childbirth remains not only a moment of profound human continuity but one of safety and empowerment.

Alexander Juusela, MD, MPH
Maternal-Fetal Medicine,
Newark Beth Israel Medical Center,
Newark, USA

Section 1

Public Health, Social Determinants, and Systemic Challenges in Labor and Delivery

Chapter 1

Maternal Morbidity and Mortality from a Population Health Perspective

Omur Cinar Elci, Sofia Beatriz Edmonson and Alexander Juusela

Abstract

Every two minutes, a woman dies due to causes related to pregnancy, labor, and delivery. In 2020, an estimated 287,000 women died, which means eight hundred women per day. The Maternal Mortality Ratio (MMR) is a litmus test that monitors the quality and outcomes of population healthcare services. Factors such as social determinants of health, healthcare delivery systems, the healthcare workforce, economic status, education, and the environment are linked to maternal morbidity and mortality. Although progress has been made globally in reducing MMR by 34% between 2000 and 2020, the disparity between the Global North and the Global South remains. The United Nations' Sustainable Development Goals (SDG) target #3.1 aims to decrease the global MMR to less than 70 maternal deaths per 100,000 live births by 2030. The current trends indicate that this target will be missed by an excess of one million preventable maternal deaths. With effective comprehensive maternal healthcare services, however, most unintended pregnancies, unsafe abortions, and maternal deaths can be eliminated. This chapter examines global maternal morbidity and mortality trends from the population health perspective, including fundamental concepts, risk factors, determinants, and proposed evidence-based solutions.

Keywords: maternal health, maternity, maternal morbidity, maternal mortality, population health, planetary health, public health, equity, social determinants of health, adolescent pregnancy, global burden of maternal health

1. Introduction

With the 2024 estimations globally, every two minutes, a woman dies due to health complications of pregnancy, labor, delivery, and other causes of maternal morbidity [1]. In 2020, around 287,000 women worldwide died due to maternal causes, which is about 800 preventable maternal deaths per day [1].

The global community has long been concerned about the high maternal morbidity and mortality and global disparity in maternal health. In 1987, the World Health Organization (WHO), the World Bank, and the United Nations Population Fund (UNFPA) organized the Safe Motherhood conference to raise global awareness of the need to reduce maternal mortality [2]. The overarching goal was to reduce maternal mortality by 50% by 2000 [2, 3]. Furthermore, in 2000, the United Nations (UN) launched the Millennium Development Goals (MDG) [4]. MDG target #5.1 aimed to reduce the maternal mortality ratio (MMR) by three-quarters, and MDG target #5.2 sought to achieve universal access to reproductive health by 2015 [4]. In 2016, the UN released the Sustainable Development Goals (SDG), which aimed to provide "a shared blueprint for peace and prosperity for people and the planet" [5]. SDG target #3.1 aims to "reduce the global MMR to less than 70 maternal deaths per 100,000 live births by 2030" [5, 6].

While considerable progress in reducing the MMR has been made, global maternal mortality remains unacceptably high, with a significant disparity between the Global North and the Global South [7]. Notably, there are success stories among countries and regions in the Global South, such as Kerala State in India [6, 8, 9], and anomalies among countries in the Global North, such as the United States (US), with a high MMR in comparison to the remaining Global North [10–12]. Strong evidence supports that most maternal mortality causes are preventable insofar as they are linked to social determinants of health (SDOH), healthcare delivery systems, the healthcare workforce, and other environmental and population factors [3, 13].

2. Fundamental concepts of maternal morbidity and mortality

One of the long-established obstacles in maternal health is the deficiency of medical understanding regarding the fundamental concepts of maternal morbidity and mortality [14]. The multilateral agencies provide adequate resources to disseminate knowledge and the relevant terminology as summarized below [15–18].

2.1 Definitions of maternal morbidity and mortality

Maternal morbidity is any short- or long-term health condition attributed to pregnancy and childbirth that has negative outcomes on the woman's well-being [15, 18, 19]. *Severe Acute Maternal Morbidity* (SAMM), also known as "near miss," refers to unintended outcomes of labor and delivery that result in significant short- or long-term consequences to maternal health, including an increased risk of maternal mortality [20].

Maternal mortality refers to the death of a woman from complications of pregnancy, childbirth, or during the postpartum period, especially the puerperium, which is the first 42 days (six weeks) of the postpartum [15, 18, 19]. *Maternal deaths* include all deaths caused or aggravated by pregnancy or childbirth-related healthcare services that occur during pregnancy or within the puerperium [17, 19]. The ICD-11 lists them under the obstetric deaths category but excludes accidental and incidental deaths [17]. The WHO defines *pregnancy-related death* as the death of a woman during pregnancy or puerperium, irrespective of the cause of death, which includes accidental and incidental causes. The US Centers for Disease Control and Prevention's (CDC) Pregnancy Mortality Surveillance System, however, defines pregnancy-related death as the death of a woman while pregnant or within 1 year of the end of a pregnancy, regardless of the outcome of the pregnancy, from any cause related to or aggravated by the pregnancy or its management, but not from an accidental or incidental cause [21]. Maternal deaths due to direct or indirect obstetric causes after the puerperium, but within less than one year of delivery, are classified by the WHO as *late maternal deaths* [17, 19]. The ICD-11 combines maternal deaths and late maternal deaths under the new category of *comprehensive maternal deaths* [6, 17].

2.2 Measures of maternal morbidity and mortality

Morbidity and mortality measures assess and monitor the natural history of maternal health problems [15, 22]. The easiest way to assess morbidity and mortality is by counting the number of cases, which provides insight into the problem's magnitude. However, counting alone is insufficient to understand the problem's scope and to compare different populations throughout time due to variations in Ref. population, data classification, or quality [15, 22].

Proportions measure the affected fraction of the population; the numerator is part of the denominator. The mid-2022 estimated population for the United Kingdom (UK) was 67,596,281, including 34,491,501 females and 33,104,780 males [23]. The proportion of the female population was 51 percent (51%) of the total population. *Ratios* measure the comparison of two subgroups of the same population. In a ratio, the numerator and the denominator are different. The female-to-male ratio in the UK is 1.04 females per male [23]. *Rates* are ratios between two quantities that have distinct units. Rates measure the change in the health problem over a specified time and reflect the risk of occurrence [15, 22]. The UK population statistics indicate that the 2022 estimated general fertility rate (GFR) is 1.75 live births per reproductive-age woman [23].

Disease morbidity measures assess the burden of diseases as the incidence or the prevalence of diseases in a defined population during a specified time. *The incidence* measures the number of new cases among people who previously did not have the disease, over the total "population-at-risk." *The prevalence* measures all cases, new and old, over the total "population-at-risk" [15, 22].

Using "*population-at-risk*" as a denominator rather than the entire population provides a more accurate morbidity estimation. Population-at-risk is the subset of the population susceptible to the disease. For example, men are not at risk of developing cervical cancer; therefore, they should be excluded from the denominator when calculating cervical cancer morbidity [15, 22]. All morbidity and mortality measures are presented with a multiplier of 1000, 10,000, 100,000, and so on to simplify the interpretation of the results [22]. For instance, the incidence rate is always presented as "per 1,000 people," and the MMR is reported as "per 100,000 live births."

Disease mortality measures assess the mortality attributed to a disease. *Mortality* is the occurrence of deaths due to a specific disease in a population at a particular time. *The mortality rate* is the number of people who died during a specified period over the total "population-at-risk" [22, 24]. Mortality rate can be calculated as a general crude rate or age, sex, and disease-specific rates. Mortality rates help compare different populations and monitor mortality data over time. These measures allow for understanding the severity trend of the disease [22]. Mortality is different from fatality.

Fatality is the occurrence of deaths due to a specific disease among those with the disease. *The Case Fatality Rate* (CFR) is the number of fatal cases over the total number of confirmed cases of the same disease during a specific time [22, 24].

The Maternal Mortality Rate (MMRate) is the number of maternal deaths in a specified period per 1000 reproductive-age women of 15–49 years during the same time [19, 22, 25].

$$\text{MMRate} = \frac{\text{number of maternal deaths}}{\text{number of reproductive age women}} \times 1{,}000$$
$$\text{at the same time}$$

The MMRate is a cause-specific mortality rate that captures the likelihood of both pregnancy and maternal deaths among women of reproductive age. Since fewer pregnancies mean fewer maternal deaths, a decrease in the MMRate may reflect a decline in fertility, even when the risk of maternal death per birth has remained constant [19, 22, 25].

The Maternal Mortality Ratio (MMR) is the number of maternal deaths during a given period per 100,000 live births during the same time [19, 22, 25].

$$\text{MMR} = \frac{\text{number of maternal deaths}}{\text{number of live births}} \times 100{,}000$$
$$\text{at the same time}$$

The MMR reflects labor and delivery-related risks. Since the MMR is not age specific, estimates from different countries are not entirely comparable. However, the MMR is still considered a litmus test of the status of women, their access to healthcare, and the adequacy of the healthcare system in responding to their needs [26]. MMR is useful in comparing the capacity of health systems to provide effective reproductive healthcare services, as well as the general health, nutrition, and degree of reproductive rights afforded to women [16]. Throughout the rest of the chapter, the MMR is reported only as a number, and it should be read as "maternal deaths per 100,000 live births."

The General Fertility Rate (GFR) is an age- and sex-specific birth rate that reflects the fertility of reproductive-age women for a specific period [19, 25]. The GFR also helps explain the relationship between the MMR and MMRate [19, 25].

$$\text{GFR} = \frac{\text{number of live births}}{\text{number of reproductive age women}} \times 1{,}000 = \frac{\text{MMRate}}{\text{MMR}}$$
$$\text{at the same time}$$

In addition to the GFR, one can calculate age-specific fertility rates for reproductive age groups of 15–19, 20–24, 25–29, 30–34, 35–39, 40–44, and 45–49 years [19, 25].

The Total Fertility Rate (TFR) is an age- and sex-adjusted birth rate that measures the average fertility of each woman until the end of reproductive age at 50 [19, 25, 27]. The TFR (Total fertility rate) is calculated as the sum of age-specific fertility rates, or five times the sum if data are given in five-year age groups, and is expressed as the number of births per woman [19, 27].

$$\text{TFR} = \frac{5}{1{,}000} \times \text{Total of Age Specific Fertility Rates}\left((15-19)+\ldots+(45-49)\right)$$

TFR is closely related to maternal and reproductive health. A TFR of 2.0 per person indicates that one woman and one man produce two children to replace themselves [27, 28]. To sustain long-term generational replacement of the population, in addition to other biological, social, and demographic factors, countries need to have a TFR of 2.1 births per person, called replacement-level fertility [29]. If the TFR exceeds 2.1, the population grows; if the TFR falls below 2.1, the population declines. The UN defines TFR above 5 births per woman as high fertility and TFR below 1.3 births per woman as very low fertility [27, 28, 30].

The lifetime risk of maternal death is the probability of a 15-year-old woman dying from maternal causes at any point during her reproductive life. The lifetime risk of maternal death can be linked to either the MMRate or the MMR [31].

$$\text{Lifetime risk of maternal death} = \text{MMRate} \times 35 = \text{MMR} \times \text{TFR}$$

The multiplier, "35," corresponds to the reproductive interval between ages 15 and 50. However, this estimation does not consider the impact of mortality risks from other causes [31].

2.3 Sources of data for measuring maternal morbidity and mortality

National and global population-based healthcare systems integrate the WHO's ICD codes into their medical recording systems to monitor all morbidities, mortalities, and health indicators [17, 19]. However, despite global efforts, measuring maternal health indicators is still a challenge, and the WHO estimates that only about 66% of actual maternal deaths are identified and classified correctly [6, 18, 32]. Due to these challenges, maternal mortality estimates are calculated using multiple data sources [17–19]. In resource-rich countries, maternal deaths are identified through routine registration of birth and death certificates. Consequently, *civil registration systems* are the main data source. *Household surveys* provide an alternative to civil registration systems. Instead of maternal deaths, these expensive surveys identify all pregnancy-related deaths [17–19]. The cost-effective version of this survey is called *the sisterhood method*, which involves researchers collecting maternal mortality data from sisters of dead women [17–19]. *Reproductive-Age Mortality Studies* (RAMOS) identify causes of maternal deaths using multiple sources of data, including civil registrations, household surveys, medical records, and death records [6, 18, 19]. They provide reliable estimates, but the process is time-consuming and expensive [6, 18, 19]. In resource-limited countries, where medical certification of the cause of death is not available, *verbal autopsies* are used to identify the cause of death from interviews with family members or members of the community [18, 19, 33]. However, unreliable data, misclassifications, and information bias are major obstacles. Finally, as a cost-effective and reliable alternative, *the national census* could produce maternal mortality estimates [19, 34].

2.4 Obstetric transition

Using the global morbidity and mortality data for 1990 and 2010, Souza et al. described a five-stage trend known as obstetric transition, in which countries gradually shift from a pattern of high maternal mortality to low maternal mortality [35]. During this transition, key changes include the aging of the maternal population, increased institutionalization of maternity care, increased obstetric interventions, and increased medicalization [35]. The most noteworthy change was the transition from direct causes to indirect causes of maternal mortality [35]. Overall, population dynamics, SDOH, access to healthcare, and the quality of care directly affected the transition between stages of the obstetrical transition.

In *stage I*, the MMR is very high, usually over 1000, along with a high fertility rate [35]. Women experience a maternal health course close to the pre-industrial, natural history of pregnancy and childbirth, without any available modern medical interventions. Hence, women with limited access to quality healthcare experience maternal deaths due primarily to direct causes [35].

In *stage II*, the MMR ranges between 300 and 999, and fertility rates remain high [35]. The causes of maternal death are usually the same as those in stage I. What differentiates countries in stage II from those in stage I is that there is some improvement in access to healthcare and increasing numbers of women seeking care at healthcare facilities [35]. In stages I and II, access to health care, healthcare facilities, workforce, education, and basic infrastructure, such as roads and transportation, are the main problems. Therefore, primordial and primary prevention are critical within the prevention services (**Figure 1**) [35, 36].

In *stage III*, although the MMR is between 50 and 299, which is still high, fertility rates vary [35]. More women have access to healthcare; however, as most deaths are still due to direct causes, healthcare quality in these countries continues to be a challenge affecting maternal mortality [35]. In Stage III, in addition to primordial and primary prevention, secondary and tertiary prevention are critical for improving maternal health outcomes [35, 36].

In *stage IV*, the MMR is moderate or low, usually less than 50, the fertility rates are low, and most maternal deaths are due to indirect causes [35]. While high utilization of medical technology is prominent, overmedication poses a threat to the quality of care, which is affected by quaternary prevention [35, 36].

In *stage V*, the MMR is less than 5, and the fertility rate is low [35]. These countries have succeeded in forestalling all preventable maternal deaths. Maternal mortality in these countries stems from indirect causes, health disparities, structural violence, and the lack of adequate care for vulnerable and marginalized communities [35]. Clinical prevention practices, especially quaternary prevention, should be emphasized in all stages of obstetric transition [36].

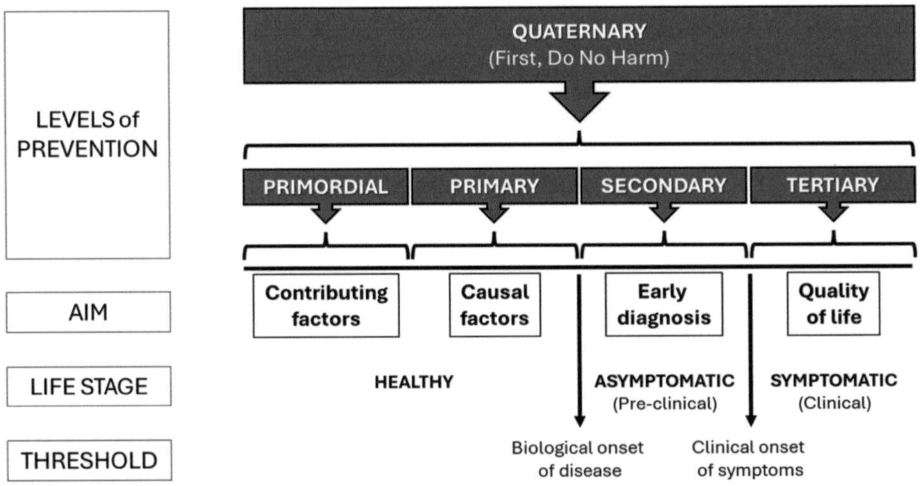

Figure 1.
Stages of prevention. Concept from Kisling and Das [36].

3. The global burden and causes of maternal morbidity and mortality

3.1 Past and present of maternal morbidity and mortality

Until the mid-1930s, the risk of maternal death in Europe was remarkably high, with an average MMR of over 500 [37–39]. Although there is limited data, globally it was estimated that as many as one in three women died, due to maternal causes, during reproductive age [40]. The common causes of maternal mortality were adolescent pregnancy, high gravidity (number of pregnancies), high parity (number of deliveries), infectious diseases, hemorrhage (bleeding), malnutrition, poor living conditions, and limited access to healthcare [38, 41]. The nineteenth-century industrial era improvements in living conditions, nutrition, and access to healthcare strengthened overall health and reduced maternal mortality [38, 41]. Although the attendance of medical practitioners at normal labor and delivery was highly regarded as a scientific advancement, it also increased the risk of post-partum infection (puerperal fever), which had a poor prognosis due to either a pelvic abscess, septicemia, or peritonitis [37, 41, 42]. In the late 1840s, Dr. Ignaz Semmelweis (1818–1865), among others, recognized that puerperal fever was a contagious and fatal disease that probably was transmitted by medical practitioners [41–43]. His proposal of hygiene, handwashing, and asepsis to prevent maternal morbidity and mortality established Dr. Semmelweis as the founder of medical hygiene and asepsis [41–43]. MMR, however, did not change much until the mid-1930s [7, 37]. The introduction of sulfonamides in the 1930s and penicillin in the 1940s led to a gradual decline in maternal mortality in Europe throughout the twentieth century [37–39, 41, 44]. However, the MMR in the Global South today continues to be a major global public health challenge [6, 45, 46].

3.2 The global burden of maternal mortality

In the analysis of the global burden of diseases, the World Bank has traditionally used Gross Domestic Product (GDP) to designate countries as low-income, middle-income, or high-income countries [47]. During the 1960s, to further highlight the impact of colonialism on the global economic divide, Oglesby devised the term "*Global South*" to identify lesser industrialized countries and former colonies in most of Africa, Asia, Latin America, the Caribbean, and Oceania [48]. "*Global North*" thus came to refer to industrialized countries and former colonial powers, including the US, Canada, European countries, Israel, the Russian Federation, Korea, Japan, Australia, and New Zealand. The UN adopted this widely used categorization in 2022 [49, 50].

Evidence-based determinants of maternal health are categorized at the individual, interpersonal, community, healthcare, and policy levels [6–8, 10, 13, 45, 46, 51–54]. Deficiencies or challenges among these factors have been detrimental to global maternal health [7, 13, 51]. At the individual level, poor education, the lack of knowledge and awareness, fear of stigma and discrimination, poverty, and financial constraints [51, 52, 54]; at the community level, SDOH, sociocultural norms, stigma, and discrimination [51, 53]; and at the healthcare and policy level, limited access to healthcare, poor quality of healthcare, inadequate infrastructure, and limited policy focus on maternal healthcare services [45, 51–56] significantly affected maternal morbidity and mortality and fueled disparity between the Global North and South. For instance, the WHO reports that while skilled birth attendants attended all births in the Global North, this proportion drops to 70% in the Global South [1]. Despite all documented determinants, most WHO policy recommendations have been vertical perspectives focused on isolated healthcare services and disease management. Global North and South countries followed these policy recommendations, expecting sustainable solutions and improvements in maternal health [1, 6, 13, 35, 57, 58]. However, limited progress has been made as the WHO policies failed to adequately emphasize the underlying SDOH, especially social justice and health equity [6, 58].

In 2000, the global MMR was 339, which translates to an annual 451,000 deaths or daily over 1200 maternal mortalities [6, 25]. Twenty years later, in 2020, the global MMR was reduced to 223, and the number of maternal deaths worldwide was around 287,000. That number represents around 800 preventable maternal deaths per day (**Figure 2**) [6, 25].

This 34.2% reduction in the global MMR between 2000 and 2020 is equivalent to a 2.1% decrease annually. Yet, progress was uneven throughout this period [6, 25]. Until 2015, the global average annual reduction rate of MMR was 2.7%. Between 2016 and 2020, this fell to −0.04% [6]. Overall, Global South countries have a higher lifetime risk of maternal death compared with those in the Global North [59]. In 2005, 99% of all maternal deaths occurred in the Global South [6, 25]. By 2020, the Global South accounted for 95% of all maternal deaths [6, 25]. In 2020, the average MMR for Sub-Saharan Africa was 545, which was 136 times higher than the MMR in Australia and New Zealand, which was 4 [6, 25, 57]. That same year, outside Sub-Saharan Africa, Afghanistan reported a very high MMR of 620, while Haiti recorded a high MMR of 350 [6, 25].

Between 2000 and 2020, 69 of the 185 countries reported a reduction in their MMR by at least half, and 34 countries reported a two-thirds reduction in their MMR [6, 25]. The top ten countries with the largest decline in their MMR between 2000 and 2020 included Belarus (95.5%), Seychelles (92.5%), Turkmenistan (80.3%), Romania (79.8%), Bhutan (79.5%), Egypt (79.0%), Estonia (79.0%), Lao People's Democratic Republic (78.7%), Kazakhstan (76.3%), and Mozambique (76.1%) [6]. In 2000, Belarus had an MMR of 24, but it succeeded in reducing this to 1 in 2020, the lowest of all countries [6]. The success story of Kerala State, in India, is also noteworthy [9, 60, 61]. In India, MMR decreased by 73.2% from 384 in 2000 to 103 in 2020, then to 97 in 2022 [6, 60, 62, 63]. However, with its 35 million population, Kerala State succeeded in reducing the MMR by over 87.3%, from 149 in 2000 to 19 in 2021, with a TFR of 1.46, which is lower than some Global North countries [6, 62, 63].

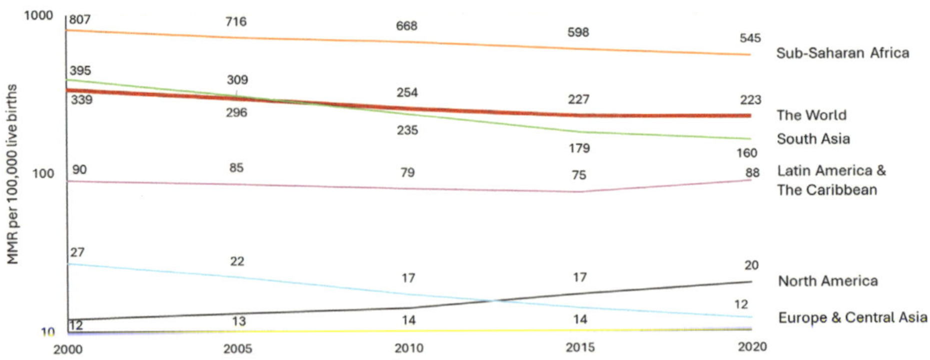

Figure 2.
Global Maternal Mortality Ratios (MMR) (2000–2020). Data from WHO [6, 25].

Ten countries saw an increase in MMR. These countries were Venezuela (−182.8%), Cyprus (−107%), Greece (−101.1%), the US (−77.9%), Mauritius (−62.1%), Puerto Rico (−55.9%), Belize (−51.3%), the Dominican Republic (−36.0%), Tonga (−32.7%), and Libya (−26.3%) [6]. Nigeria had the highest estimated number of maternal deaths, accounting for 28.5% of all estimated global maternal deaths in 2020 [6]. North America has experienced an increase in MMR from 12 in 2000 to 21 in 2020, mostly due to increasing MMR in the US [6, 25]. Among the Global North countries, the US had the highest MMR, with 21 in 2020, which has increased by 77.9% since 2000 [6]. The CDC Pregnancy Mortality Surveillance System reported that the MMR further increased to 32.9 overall and 69.9 for Black American women in 2021 [64, 65].

The global lifetime risk of maternal mortality for a 15-year-old girl in 2020 was estimated at 1 in 210, approximately half the risk faced by a 15-year-old girl in 2000 [6]. In 2020, a 15-year-old girl in Sub-Saharan Africa had a 1 in 40 chance of maternal death, which is approximately 400 times higher than a 15-year-old girl in Australia and New Zealand, where the lifetime risk is 1 in 16,000 [6].

Total fertility is closely related to maternal health. Between 1950 and 2021, global TFR more than halved, from 4.84 to 2.23 births per woman [29]. According to estimates from the 2021 Global Burden of Disease Study, the global TFR will drop to 1.83 births per woman in 2050 and 1.59 births per woman in 2100. While the TFR will drop significantly in the Global North, most of the global live births in 2100 will occur in the Global South. These changes will have major socioeconomic consequences globally [29].

The MMR trend over two decades suggests that even though most maternal deaths occur in Global South countries, the status of a country as a Global North or Global South is not the only determining factor of a country's progress in addressing maternal health challenges. Given current trends, the global MMR for 2030 is projected to be around 222 maternal deaths per 100,000 live births, which is more than three times the SDG target #3.1 [6]. This means that the SDG target will be missed by an excess of 1 million additional preventable maternal deaths [6].

3.3 Top causes of global maternal morbidity and mortality

Maternal deaths have been categorized as having direct or indirect causes [6, 19, 66]. *Direct maternal deaths* are those caused by pregnancy, labor, and puerperium-related complications [6, 19, 66]. *Indirect maternal deaths* are caused by pre-existing medical conditions or by diseases developed during pregnancy, which may be aggravated by the physiological effects of pregnancy [66–68]. Direct and indirect causes can be interconnected. For example, unsafe medical practices can lead to hemorrhage or postpartum infections, which are direct causes [69]. In turn, postpartum infections can increase the risk of thromboembolism [70], and hemorrhage can lead to or exacerbate anemia, which is an indirect cause of maternal mortality [69–71].

In 2014 the WHO reported that between 2003 and 2009, the top causes of maternal deaths globally were HIV-related diseases (27.5%), hemorrhage (27.1%), hypertensive disorders in pregnancy (14.0%), pregnancy-related infections/sepsis (10.7%), other direct causes of death (9.6%), pregnancy termination complications (7.9%), and embolism (3.2%) [71]. In 2023, the top causes of maternal mortality were reported to be non-obstetric complications (48.32%), hemorrhage (17.63%), hypertensive disorders in pregnancy (14.01%), other obstetric complications (7.11%), pregnancy termination (5.41%), pregnancy-related infection (5.26%), and unanticipated complications of obstetric management (2.25%) [57].

There are, however, observed differences in country- and region-specific causal factors. Between 2017 and 2019, the top causes of maternal morbidity and mortality in the US were mental health disorders, which include depression, substance abuse, and suicide (22.7%); cardiovascular disorders (21.3%); hemorrhage (13.7%); pulmonary and amniotic embolisms (12.5%); infections (9.2%); hypertensive disorders (6.5%); injury (3.6%); cerebrovascular disorders (2.5%); cancer (1.9%), metabolic/endocrine disorders (1.2%); and pulmonary disorders (1.2%) [72]. Mental health-related MMRate in the US also varied with 7.7% among Asian women, 8.6% among Black women, and 36.4% among White women [21]. Each demographic may require a tailored approach to understanding and addressing the unique factors influencing maternal health outcomes. Between 2015 and 2020, the leading causes of death in Sub-Saharan African countries were hemorrhage (28.8%), hypertensive disorders in pregnancy (22.1%), non-obstetric complications (18.8%), and pregnancy-related infections/sepsis (11.5%) [73]. Besides geographic location and country, various sociodemographic characteristics, such as maternal age, education, health disparities, and other factors, have been investigated for their role in maternal morbidity and mortality [74].

3.3.1 Direct causes of maternal morbidity and mortality

Globally, hemorrhage, pregnancy-related infections, and hypertensive disorders are the top three direct causes of maternal morbidity and mortality, accounting for 51.9% of all maternal deaths [71]. In addition, direct causes, including obstetrical complications and unsafe pregnancy terminations, account for nearly 75% of all maternal deaths [1].

3.3.1.1 Hemorrhage

The WHO recognizes hemorrhage as the leading cause of maternal mortality around the world [71, 75]. Of the 14 million women globally who experience postpartum hemorrhage annually, about 70,000 die as a result, mostly in the Global South [75, 76]. The majority of postpartum hemorrhage cases occur due to uterine atony, genital tract lacerations, or the retention of placental tissue [57, 75–79]. Although the risk of postpartum hemorrhage is relatively low in the US, the risk is not uniformly distributed throughout the US population [76]. White women have a lower risk of postpartum hemorrhage compared to Black and Indigenous women in the US, which reflects the maternal health disparity [80, 81].

3.3.1.2 Infections

Pregnancy-related infections are among the most common causes of maternal mortality because they increase the risk of sepsis [71, 82]. The Pan American Health Organization (PAHO) estimates that 11 out of 1000 pregnant women experience infection-related severe organ dysfunction or death [83]. The most common sources of maternal infections were the genital tract, urinary tract, skin or soft tissue, and respiratory tract [84, 85]. The WHO and Jhpiego, an affiliate of Johns Hopkins University, launched the Global Maternal and Neonatal Sepsis Initiative in 2017 to reduce preventable maternal and neonatal deaths from sepsis. Jhpiego aims to boost "maternal health providers' skills and develop systems that save lives." [82, 86].

3.3.1.3 Hypertensive disorders

Hypertensive disorders in pregnancy include chronic hypertension, gestational hypertension, pre-eclampsia/eclampsia, chronic hypertension complicated with preeclampsia/eclampsia, and HELLP (hemolysis, elevated liver enzymes, and low platelet count) syndrome [87, 88]. Globally, between 5% and 10% of pregnant women experience hypertension during pregnancy [87, 89]. Between 1990 and 2020, the global incidence of hypertensive disorders in pregnancy increased by 10.9%, from 16.3 million to 18.1 million [88]. There was, however, a 30.1% decrease in mortality due to hypertensive disorders in pregnancy. Most of those deaths occurred in the Global South among women who were 25–29 years of age [88].

3.3.2 Indirect causes of maternal morbidity and mortality

Similar to direct causes, the highest number of cases of indirect maternal morbidity and mortality occur in the Global South countries where maternal morbidity and mortality are attributed to infectious diseases, including HIV disease, malaria, and tuberculosis, as well as to non-communicable diseases such as anemia, diabetes mellitus, respiratory diseases, and cardiovascular conditions [66–68].

3.3.2.1 HIV disease

In 2022, globally, there were 1.2 million pregnant women with HIV [1]. Most of these women live in the Global South, especially in Sub-Saharan Africa. Pregnant women with HIV face significant challenges that contribute to an elevated maternal mortality of 2 to 10 times higher than those without the infection [90]. In regions where the prevalence of HIV among pregnant women is 2%, it is estimated that 12% of all maternal deaths are attributable to HIV [91]. HIV-related indirect maternal deaths accounted for about 2% of all maternal deaths in 2005. As progress has been made in tackling the HIV pandemic, HIV disease accounted for less than 1% of all maternal deaths in 2020 [6]. Still, in many Sub-Saharan African countries, HIV disease is among the leading causes of maternal morbidity and mortality [67, 68]. HIV increases the risk of opportunistic infections due to decreased CD4 T helper cells, which are responsible for helping fight these infections. Thus, HIV disease can raise the risk of pregnancy complications both directly through disease progression and indirectly through postpartum infections and increased risk of tuberculosis [67, 68].

3.3.2.2 Anemia

In 2020, an estimated 38% of pregnant women suffered from anemia globally [68, 92]. While 22% of women in the Global North have anemia, in the Global South, 56% of women have anemia [92]. Poor nutrition is among the most prevalent causes of anemia, especially iron deficiency anemia [93, 94]. Malaria and HIV disease can also lead to anemia [68, 95]. Regardless of the cause, anemia can increase the risk of postpartum hemorrhage [96]. Severe pregnancy-related hemorrhage also increases the severity of anemia and the risk of hemorrhagic fatalities or anemia-induced heart failure [96, 97].

3.3.2.3 Malaria

Malaria, especially severe malaria, increases maternal mortality [95, 98]. The WHO defines severe malaria as either (a) hemoglobin of less than 7 g/dL or hematocrit of less than 20% with a parasite count of more than 10,000/μL, or (b) hyperparasitemia, which is defined as an infection of 10% or more of the red blood cells [95, 98]. In 2020, the risk of maternal death among women with severe malaria in Southeast Asia was estimated at 12.2% [95, 98]. When malaria is coupled with either hypotension, respiratory failure, or coma, which are signs of end-organ damage, the CFR is about 29.1% [95, 98]. In countries where malaria is prevalent, given its damage to red blood cells, it is not uncommon for pregnant women in labor to be found to have hemoglobin levels below 5 g/dL, which is considered severe anemia [99].

4. High-risk groups in maternal morbidity and mortality

The global disparity in maternal morbidity and mortality becomes more prominent among minority, disadvantaged, and marginalized women [6, 25, 100]. In many countries, simply being a woman is a high morbidity and mortality risk due to patriarchal cultural practices where the health and welfare of men are often prioritized [100]. Women, especially pregnant women, may be further at risk due to many factors, including their race, ethnicity, education, SDOH, refugee or migrant status, and being incarcerated.

4.1 Women in poverty

Poverty does not occur naturally or in isolation; socioeconomic systems, policies, disparities, and the lack of social justice directly affect health and create an uneven, unjust climate for populations, especially for women [58]. Poverty causes a loop of disparities in access to education, healthcare, work, healthy living opportunities, and a safe environment, all of which directly affect maternal health [58, 101]. Globally, the poorest and least educated women are the most susceptible to maternal morbidity and mortality [13]. Poverty affects the quality and access to healthcare services and access to trained healthcare practitioners [100–102]. Poverty further increases systemic racism, health disparities, and related disproportional high maternal mortality [102–105]. Moreover, women in poverty face higher rates of incarceration, substance abuse, mental health conditions, chronic medical conditions, and limited access to healthcare, all of which further deteriorate maternal health outcomes for women in poverty [106].

4.2 Refugees and migrant women

Refugees and migrant women face serious maternal health challenges due to marginalization, discrimination, cultural differences, limited access to healthcare, and socioeconomic instability [107–109]. Compared to native-born women, migrant or refugee women in the Global North have a higher risk of adverse maternal outcomes unless they are from Europe, the Middle East, or North Africa [109]. Therefore, racism or discrimination against certain cultural differences may trigger major maternal health disparities [107–109].

4.3 Racial and ethnic minority women

A closer examination of the unusually high MMR in the US [6, 64] reveals that Black and Indigenous women have significantly higher maternal morbidity and mortality [10, 104, 105, 110–112]. According to the CDC, in 2021, the MMR for Black women increased to 69.9 compared to 28.0 for Latina and 26.6 for White women [64]. Around 75% of Black pregnant women in the US are treated by only 25% of hospitals, mostly in urban areas [111]. Besides social disparities, the high cost of healthcare, discrimination, systemic racism, and poor access to healthcare affect maternal morbidity and mortality among minority women [101, 113, 114]. Racism-induced chronic stress has been associated with an increased risk of co-morbidities, epigenetic changes, and a higher risk of hypertension and cardiovascular disease as the major causes of maternal morbidity and mortality [101]. As Dr. Joia Crear-Perry states, "Race is not a factor for illness and death, but racism, bias, and discrimination are [113]."

4.4 Women with physical disabilities

Studies report that women with physical, sensory, or intellectual impairment or disabilities have an 11 times higher risk of maternal mortality compared to non-disabled women, four times the risk for heart problems, about three times the risk for infection, and more than double the risk for severe preeclampsia and placenta previa [115, 116].

4.5 Adolescent and advanced-aged mothers

Although the global adolescent birth rate has decreased from 64.5 births per 1000 women in 2000 to 41.3 in 2023, the WHO estimates that 21 million girls between 15 and 19 years of age, mostly from the Global South, become pregnant annually [117]. Compared to Europe, where the adolescent birth rate is 13.1 births per 1000 women, the adolescent birth rate is higher in Latin America and the Caribbean, with 51.4, and in Sub-Saharan Africa, with 97.9 [117, 118]. Adolescent mothers are at greater risk of experiencing eclampsia, puerperal and systemic infections, sexually transmitted infections, anemia, pregnancy-related hypertension, and premature deliveries compared to 20–24-year-old women [117, 118]. Women over 35 are also at higher risk of pregnancy loss, ectopic pregnancy, gestational hypertension, gestational diabetes, prolonged labor, and genetic disorders [118, 119].

5. Proposed solutions to reduce maternal morbidity and mortality

Global evidence showed that effective social interventions and integrated comprehensive healthcare services can prevent 68% of unintended pregnancies, 72% of unsafe abortions, and 62% of maternal deaths [1, 120]. Integrated, evidence-based, population-focused healthcare interventions can produce sustainable and effective solutions to improve maternal health [51, 53, 55, 121–123]. Focusing on the SDOH, eliminating health disparities, improving healthcare services, ensuring universal coverage for comprehensive primary care, addressing all causes of maternal morbidity and mortality, and strengthening health systems to collect high-quality data are important steps in improving maternal health globally [1, 13]. Interventions to improve healthcare services in all six dimensions of healthcare, including accessibility, availability, acceptability, affordability, accommodation, and awareness, affect maternal health outcomes directly [51, 53]. As we noted, contrary to these recommendations, vertical-focused WHO policy recommendations, which neglected the underlying SDOH, especially social justice and health equity, delivered limited progress in maternal health globally [1, 6, 13, 35, 57, 58]. Therefore, comprehensive, integrated, accessible, available, acceptable, affordable, and accommodating primary healthcare services with awareness and effective coverage are fundamental in promoting maternal health [51–53, 55, 58, 121–123]. Sustainability and success would come with integrating healthcare services with population-focused, socially and culturally sensitive interventions, such as poverty reduction interventions, family and peer support programs, women's education and empowerment, mental health support, and training [51, 53, 122]. Although health literacy and social and behavioral change intervention programs may add value to the success of maternal health services, it was demonstrated that vertical, isolated programs without integration into population-based social, cultural, and healthcare interventions do not reduce maternal morbidity and mortality [55, 122, 124]. Integrating traditional healers with primary healthcare services in rural settings of the Global South and establishing community education programs to eliminate stigma and discrimination—including the stigma surrounding mental health—have been effective in promoting maternal health [53, 121]. However, in the case of the US, where the maternal health indicators are abnormally poor, implementation of isolated measures such as doula programs, or focusing on healthcare coverage alone, would be insufficient [55, 125, 126]. Examining evidence and revisiting determinants of obstetric transition demonstrates that resolving maternal health challenges in the US will require more comprehensive, systematic healthcare reform starting from state to federal level, integrated with population-based, social, and financial system changes [35, 126].

Nobel laureate Amartya Sen described health equity as a central feature of social justice [127]. He argues that health equity must be analyzed concurrently with fairness and justice in social systems, including wealth distribution and freedom. Therefore, tackling maternal health challenges requires a vision beyond health outcomes to encompass planetary capability by eliminating economic disparities, systemic racism, and neo-colonial policies and addressing unjust social arrangements within and beyond healthcare systems [56, 127, 128]. All countries that have successfully reduced maternal mortality have focused on human potential instead of economic indicators. Countries and states such as Belarus or Kerala State in India established population-based, community-oriented primary healthcare services to provide equitable, accessible, integrated services, including maternal and child healthcare [9, 61, 103]. The Kerala Development Model's success since the 1970s relied on government investments in health and education, women's empowerment, integrated health literacy, social mobilization, labor organizations, and community participation programs [9, 61]. Women's and their partners' education directly affects the utilization of maternal healthcare services and health outcomes [102, 129, 130].

Sustainable success in maternal and reproductive health will be possible only if policymakers measure development using human well-being rather than GDP per capita or other economic indicators. A sustainable approach to current maternal health challenges demands a social justice and equity-focused paradigm change, including fundamental progressive transformation, new economic and social policies, and inclusive science and technology interventions. Health, as a human right, cannot stand alone without a peaceful and prosperous global society that needs equitable decision-making power shared by all.

Acknowledgements

As the authors, we appreciate the assistance and support of Alicia Oliver, MD, MPH, who helped with the literature search and contributed to the early drafts of the manuscript. We also thank Professor Namik Demir, MD, John M. Okoye, MD, and Onder Bayata, MD, who served as peer reviewers. Their valuable notes improved the depth and content of the manuscript.

Author details

Omur Cinar Elci[1*], Sofia Beatriz Edmonson[1] and Alexander Juusela[2]

1 Western Atlantic University School of Medicine, Freeport, The Bahamas

2 Newark Beth Israel Medical Center, New Jersey, USA

*Address all correspondence to: oelci@wausm.education

References

[1] The World Health Organization (WHO). Maternal mortality. WHO. Available from: https://www.who.int/news-room/fact-sheets/detail/maternal-mortality [Accessed: June 4, 2024]

[2] Mahler H. The safe motherhood initiative: A call to action. Lancet. 1987;**1**(8534); Art. no. 8534. DOI: 10.1016/s0140-6736(87)90423-5

[3] Nour NM. An introduction to maternal mortality. Reviews in Obstetrics and Gynecology. 2008;**1**(2):77-81

[4] Migiro A-R. The importance of the MDGs: The United Nations leadership in development. United Nations. Available from: https://www.un.org/en/chronicle/article/importance-mdgs-united-nations-leadership-development [Accessed: June 14, 2024]

[5] The United Nations (UN). Transforming our world: The 2030 agenda for sustainable development | Department of economic and social affairs. Available from: https://sdgs.un.org/2030agenda [Accessed: July 3, 2024]

[6] The World Health Organization (WHO), United Nations International Children's Emergency Fund (UNICEF), and United Nations Population Fund (UNFPA). Trends in maternal mortality 2000 to 2020. Available from: https://www.who.int/publications-detail-redirect/9789240068759 [Accessed: June 4, 2024]

[7] Boerma T et al. Maternal mortality, stillbirths, and neonatal mortality: A transition model based on analyses of 151 countries. The Lancet Global Health. 2023;**11**(7):e1024-e1031. DOI: 10.1016/S2214-109X(23)00195-X

[8] Campbell OMR, Amouzou A, Blumenberg C, Boerma T. Learning from success: The main drivers of the maternal and newborn health transition in seven positive-outlier countries and implications for future policies and programmes. BMJ Global Health. 2024;**9**(Suppl 2):e012126. DOI: 10.1136/bmjgh-2023-012126

[9] Krishnan A et al. Re-engineering primary healthcare in Kerala. Public Health Action. 2023;**13**(Suppl. 1): 19-25. Art. no. Suppl 1. DOI: 10.5588/pha.22.0033

[10] Cho J, Chien L-C, Holditch-Davis D. Sociodemographic and biological factors of health disparities of mothers and their very low birth-weight infants. Advances in Neonatal Care. 2022;**22**(5); Art. no. 5. DOI: 10.1097/ANC.0000000000000997

[11] Joseph KS et al. Maternal mortality in the United States: Are the high and rising rates due to changes in obstetrical factors, maternal medical conditions, or maternal mortality surveillance? American Journal of Obstetrics and Gynecology. 2024;**230**(4):440.e1-440.e13. DOI: 10.1016/j.ajog.2023.12.038

[12] Trost S, Busacker A, Leonard M. Pregnancy-related deaths: Data from maternal mortality review committees in 38 U.S. states, 2020. CDC Maternal Mortality Prevention. 2024. Available from: https://www.cdc.gov/maternal-mortality/php/data-research/index.html [Accessed: July 1, 2024]

[13] Souza JP et al. A global analysis of the determinants of maternal health and transitions in maternal mortality. The Lancet Global Health. 2024;**12**(2):e306-e316. DOI: 10.1016/S2214-109X(23)00468-0

[14] New York Academy of Medicine. Postgraduate medical education-with especial reference to present maternal mortality rates in the United States. Bulletin of the New York Academy of Medicine. 1937;**13**(10); Art. no. 10

[15] Bonita R, Beaglehole R, Kjellström T, WHO. Basic Epidemiology. World Health Organization (WHO); 2006. Available from: https://iris.who.int/handle/10665/43541 [Accessed: June 4, 2024]

[16] The United Nations (UN). Population division, "World Fertility Data". Available from: https://www.un.org/development/desa/pd/data/world-fertility-data [Accessed: June 14, 2024]

[17] The World Health Organization (WHO). ICD-11. Available from: https://icd.who.int/en [Accessed: June 14, 2024]

[18] The World Health Organization (WHO), World Bank, The United Nations Population Fund (UNFPA), and The United Nations Children's Fund (UNICEF). Maternal Mortality in 2005. Geneva, Switzerland: WHO. p. 40

[19] The World Health Organization (WHO). WHO guidance for measuring maternal mortality from a census. Available from: https://www.who.int/publications/i/item/9789241506113 [Accessed: June 14, 2024]

[20] ACOG. Obstetric care consensus No. 5: Severe maternal morbidity: Screening and review. Obstetrics and Gynecology. 2016;**128**(3):e54-e60. DOI: 10.1097/AOG.0000000000001642

[21] The Centers for Disease Control and Prevention (CDC). Pregnancy mortality surveillance system maternal mortality prevention. Available from: https://www.cdc.gov/maternal-mortality/php/pregnancy-mortality-surveillance/index.html [Accessed: July 1, 2024]

[22] Celentano DD, Szklo M. Gordis Epidemiology. 6th ed. Amsterdam: Elsevier; 2018

[23] United Kingdom Office for National Statistics. The UK Population estimates. Census. 2021. Available from: https://www.ons.gov.uk/peoplepopulationandcommunity/populationandmigration/populationestimates [Accessed: June 12, 2024]

[24] Rasmussen S, Goodman R. The CDC Field Epidemiology Manual. Oxford University Press; 2018. Available from: https://www.cdc.gov/eis/field-epi-manual/index.html [Accessed: June 4, 2024]

[25] The United Nations International Children's Emergency Fund (UNICEF). Maternal mortality rates and statistics. Available from: https://data.unicef.org/topic/maternal-health/maternal-mortality/ [Accessed: June 4, 2024]

[26] The United Nations (UN). Maternal mortality figures substantially underestimated, New WHO/UNICEF Study Says | Meetings Coverage and Press Releases. Available from: https://press.un.org/en/1996/19960205.h2896.html [Accessed: June 4, 2024]

[27] Moran A. What factors affect the Total fertility rate, or TFR? Population Education. 2020. Available from: https://populationeducation.org/what-factors-affect-the-total-fertility-rate-or-tfr/ [Accessed: June 26, 2024]

[28] Fauser BCJM et al. Declining global fertility rates and the implications for family planning and family building: An IFFS consensus document based on a narrative review of the literature. Human

Reproduction Update. 2024;**30**(2):2. DOI: 10.1093/humupd/dmad028

[29] Bhattacharjee NV et al. Global fertility in 204 countries and territories, 1950-2021, with forecasts to 2100: A comprehensive demographic analysis for the global burden of disease study 2021. The Lancet. 2024;**403**(10440); Art. no. 10440. DOI: 10.1016/S0140-6736(24)00550-6

[30] The United Nations (UN). Total fertility rate. 2007. Available from: https://www.un.org/esa/sustdev/natlinfo/indicators/methodology_sheets/demographics/total_fertility_rate.pdf [Accessed: July 5, 2024]

[31] Wilmoth J. The lifetime risk of maternal mortality: Concept and measurement. Bulletin of the World Health Organization. 2009;**87**(4):256-262. Art. no. 4. DOI: 10.2471/BLT.07.048280

[32] Ahmed SMA, Cresswell JA, Say L. Incompleteness and misclassification of maternal death recording: A systematic review and meta-analysis. BMC Pregnancy and Childbirth. 2023;**23**(1):794-810. Art. no. 1. DOI: 10.1186/s12884-023-06077-4

[33] The World Health Organization (WHO). Verbal autopsy standards: Ascertaining and attributing causes of death tool. CC BY-ND 3.0 IGO, 2022. Available from: https://www.who.int/standards/classifications/other-classifications/verbal-autopsy-standards-ascertaining-and-attributing-causes-of-death-tool [Accessed: July 1, 2024]

[34] The US Census Bureau. Measuring maternal mortality. Census.gov. Available from: https://www.census.gov/programs-surveys/international-programs/events/training/select-topics-in-international-censuses/questionnaire/maternal-mortality.html [Accessed: July 1, 2024]

[35] Souza J et al. Obstetric transition: The pathway towards ending preventable maternal deaths. BJOG: An International Journal of Obstetrics & Gynaecology. 2014;**121**(s1):1-4. Art. no. s1. DOI: 10.1111/1471-0528.12735

[36] Kisling LA, Das JM. Prevention strategies. In: StatPearls. Treasure Island (FL): StatPearls Publishing; 2024. Available from: http://www.ncbi.nlm.nih.gov/books/NBK537222/ [Accessed: July 31, 2024]

[37] Loudon I. Deaths in childbed from the eighteenth century to 1935. Medical History. 1986;**30**(1):1-41. Art. no. 1

[38] Reid A. The geography of maternal mortality in early twentieth century England and Wales. Annales de Demographie Historique. 2020;**139**(1):111-140. Art. no. 1

[39] Hanson C. Data on maternal mortality. 2010. Available from: https://www.gapminder.org/documentation/documentation/gapdoc010.pdf [Accessed: July 8, 2024]

[40] Reid A. How dangerous was childbirth in the past? In: The Cambridge Group for the History of Population and Social Structure. Cambridge. Available from: https://www.campop.geog.cam.ac.uk/blog/2024/09/19/childbirth-in-the-past/ [Accessed: February 14, 2025]

[41] Chamberlain G. British maternal mortality in the 19th and early 20th centuries. Journal of the Royal Society of Medicine. 2006;**99**(11):559-563. Art. no. 11

[42] Carter KC. Puerperal Fever. In: Kiple KF, editor. The Cambridge

World History of Human Disease. Cambridge: Cambridge University Press; 1993. pp. 955-957. DOI: 10.1017/CHOL9780521332866.175

[43] Kadar N, Romero R, Papp Z. Ignaz Semmelweis: 'The savior of mothers' on the 200th anniversary of the birth. American Journal of Obstetrics and Gynecology. 2018;**219**(6):519-522. Art. no. 6. DOI: 10.1016/j.ajog.2018.10.036

[44] Colebrook L, Kenny M, The members of the Honorary Staff of Queen Charlotte's Hospital. Treatment with prontosil of puerperal infections: Due to haemolytic streptococci. The Lancet. 1936;**228**(5910):1319-1322. Art. no. 5910. DOI: 10.1016/S0140-6736(00)48180-8

[45] Ekwuazi EK, Chigbu CO, Ngene NC. Reducing maternal mortality in low- and middle-income countries. Case Reports in Women's Health. 2023;**39**:e00542. DOI: 10.1016/j.crwh.2023.e00542

[46] Lawrence ER, Klein TJ, Beyuo TK. Maternal mortality in low and middle-income countries. Obstetrics and Gynecology Clinics of North America. 2022;**49**(4):713-733. Art. no. 4. DOI: 10.1016/j.ogc.2022.07.001

[47] Fleming S. The World Bank's 2020 country classifications explained. World Economic Forum. Available from: https://www.weforum.org/agenda/2020/08/world-bank-2020-classifications-low-high-income-countries/ [Accessed: June 18, 2024]

[48] Hogan E, Patrick S. A closer look at the global south. Carnegie endowment for international peace. Available from: https://carnegieendowment.org/research/2024/05/global-south-colonialism-imperialism?lang=en [Accessed: June 18, 2024]

[49] The United Nations (UN). General assembly takes up second committee reports, Adopting 38 resolutions, 2 decisions. UN Press Release GA/12482. Available from: https://press.un.org/en/2022/ga12482.doc.htm [Accessed: June 18, 2024]

[50] Hossain S. 'Third World' or 'Global South'? It's time to redefine. South Asia Monitor. Available from: https://www.southasiamonitor.org/perspective/third-world-or-global-south-its-time-redefine [Accessed: June 18, 2024]

[51] Yihune Teshale M, Bante A, Gedefaw Belete A, Crutzen R, Spigt M, Stutterheim SE. Barriers and facilitators to maternal healthcare in East Africa: A systematic review and qualitative synthesis of perspectives from women, their families, healthcare providers, and key stakeholders. BMC Pregnancy and Childbirth. 2025;**25**(1):111. DOI: 10.1186/s12884-025-07225-8

[52] Ali N, Philip S, Vishnoi R, Deepika. A narrative review on the effectiveness of interventions promoting antenatal care proficiency in terms of knowledge, attitude, and practice maternal wellness made better. International Journal of Gynecology & Obstetrics. 2025;**7**(1):15-18. DOI: 10.33545/26642298.2025.v7.i1a.178

[53] Morgan J, Breau GM. Access to maternal health services for indigenous women in low- and middle-income countries: An updated integrative review of the literature from 2018 to 2023. Rural and Remote Health. 2024;**24**(2):8520-8532. DOI: 10.22605/RRH8520

[54] Singh R, Singh H, Singh A, Prashar N, Lachyan A. Advancing maternal and child health: A comprehensive analysis of United Nations' sustainable development goals. Majmaah Journal of Health Sciences.

2025;**13**(1):88-88. DOI: 10.5455/mjhs.2025.01.009

[55] Kassie AM, Eakin E, Endalamaw A, Zewdie A, Wolka E, Assefa Y. Effective coverage of maternal and neonatal healthcare services in low-and middle-income countries: A scoping review. BMC Health Services Research. 2024;**24**:1601. DOI: 10.1186/s12913-024-12085-7

[56] Sundari TK. The untold story: How the health Care Systems in Developing Countries Contribute to maternal mortality. International Journal of Health Services: Planning, Administration, Evaluation. 1992;**22**(3):513-528. Art. no. 3. DOI: 10.2190/91YH-A52T-AFBB-1LEA

[57] Alipour J, Payandeh A, Karimi A. Prevalence of maternal mortality causes based on ICD-MM: A systematic review and meta-analysis. BMC Pregnancy and Childbirth. 2023;**23**:821. DOI: 10.1186/s12884-023-06142-y

[58] Kwete X et al. Decolonizing global health: What should be the target of this movement and where does it lead us? Global Health Research and Policy. 2022;**7**(1):3. DOI: 10.1186/s41256-022-00237-3

[59] Sims DA. When I say ... global south and global north. Medical Education. 2024;**58**(3):286-287. Art. no. 3. DOI: 10.1111/medu.15263

[60] Ministry of Women and Child Development. Significant decline in maternal mortality in India. Available from: http://pib.gov.in/FeaturesDeatils.aspx?NoteId=151238 [Accessed: July 11, 2024]

[61] Muraleedharan M, Chandak AO. Emerging challenges in the health systems of Kerala, India: Qualitative analysis of literature reviews. Journal of Health Research. 2021;**36**(2):242-254. DOI: 10.1108/JHR-04-2020-0091

[62] Balsarkar G. Mothers shouldn't die: Significant decline in maternal mortality in India. Journal of Obstetrics and Gynecology of India. 2023;**73**(2):99-101. Art. no. 2. DOI: 10.1007/s13224-023-01754-y

[63] Meh C et al. Trends in maternal mortality in India over two decades in nationally representative surveys. BJOG. 2022;**129**(4):550-561. Art. no. 4. DOI: 10.1111/1471-0528.16888

[64] D. L. Hoyert. Maternal mortality rates in the United States, 2021. CDC Health E-Stats; 2023. Available from: https://www.cdc.gov/nchs/data/hestat/maternal-mortality/2021/maternal-mortality-rates-2021.htm

[65] Khalil A, Samara A, O'Brien P, Coutinho CM, Quintana SM, Ladhani SN. A call to action: The global failure to effectively tackle maternal mortality rates. The Lancet Global Health. 2023;**11**(8):e1165-e1167. Art. no. 8. DOI: 10.1016/S2214-109X(23)00247-4

[66] Hossain N, Shaikh ZF. Maternal deaths due to indirect causes: Report from a tertiary care center of a developing country. Obstetric Medicine. 2022;**15**(3):176-179. Art. no. 3. DOI: 10.1177/1753495X211037916

[67] Storm F, Agampodi S, Eddleston M, Sørensen JB, Konradsen F, Rheinländer T. Indirect causes of maternal death. The Lancet Global Health. 2014;**2**(10):e566. Art. no. 10. DOI: 10.1016/S2214-109X(14)70297-9

[68] Nair M, Nelson-Piercy C, Knight M. Indirect maternal deaths: UK and global perspectives. Obstetric Medicine. 2017;**10**(1):10-15. Art. no. 1. DOI: 10.1177/1753495X16689444

[69] The World Health Organization (WHO). Abortion. Available from: https://www.who.int/news-room/fact-sheets/detail/abortion [Accessed: June 7, 2024]

[70] Shirazi M, Sahebdel B, Torkzaban M, Feizabad E, Ghaemi M. Maternal mortality following thromboembolism; incidences and prophylaxis strategies. Thrombosis Journal. 2020;**18**(1): 36-43. Art. no. 1. DOI: 10.1186/s12959-020-00251-w

[71] Say L et al. Global causes of maternal death: A WHO systematic analysis. The Lancet Global Health. 2014;**2**(6):e323-e333. Art. no. 6. DOI: 10.1016/S2214-109X(14)70227-X

[72] Trost S et al. Pregnancy-related deaths: Data from maternal mortality review committees in 36 U.S. states, 2017-2019. CDC Maternal Mortality Prevention. 2022. Available from: https://www.cdc.gov/maternal-mortality/php/data-research/mmrc-2017-2019.html [Accessed: June 26, 2024]

[73] Musarandega R, Nyakura M, Machekano R, Pattinson R, Munjanja SP. Causes of maternal mortality in sub-Saharan Africa: A systematic review of studies published from 2015 to 2020. Journal of Global Health. 2021;**11**:04048. DOI: 10.7189/jogh.11.04048

[74] Neal S et al. The causes of maternal mortality in adolescents in low and middle income countries: A systematic review of the literature. BMC Pregnancy and Childbirth. 2016;**16**:352. DOI: 10.1186/s12884-016-1120-8

[75] The World Health Organization (WHO). Postpartum haemorrhage. Available from: https://www.who.int/teams/sexual-and-reproductive-health-and-research-(srh)/areas-of-work/maternal-and-perinatal-health/postpartum-haemorrhage [Accessed: June 5, 2024]

[76] The World Health Organization (WHO). A Roadmap to combat postpartum haemorrhage between 2023 and 2030. Sexual and Reproductive Health and Research (SRH). Available from: https://www.who.int/publications/i/item/9789240081802 [Accessed: June 5, 2024]

[77] Gill P, Patel A, Van Hook JW. Uterine atony. In: StatPearls. Treasure Island (FL): StatPearls Publishing; 2024. Available from: http://www.ncbi.nlm.nih.gov/books/NBK493238/ [Accessed: June 5, 2024]

[78] Jones AJ, Federspiel JJ, Eke AC. Preventing postpartum hemorrhage with combined therapy rather than oxytocin alone. American Journal of Obstetrics & Gynecology MFM. 2023;**5**(2):100731-100743. Supplement, Art. no. 2, Supplement. DOI: 10.1016/j.ajogmf.2022.100731

[79] The World Health Organization (WHO). WHO recommendations for the prevention of postpartum haemorrhage. 2007. Available from: https://www.afro.who.int/sites/default/files/2017-06/WHO_MPS_0706_engPPH.pdf [Accessed: June 30, 2024]

[80] Gyamfi-Bannerman C et al. Postpartum hemorrhage outcomes and race. American Journal of Obstetrics and Gynecology. 2018;**219**(2):185.e1-185.e10. Art. no. 2. DOI: 10.1016/j.ajog.2018.04.052

[81] Okunlola O et al. Race/ethnicity as a risk factor in the development of postpartum hemorrhage: A thorough systematic review of disparity in the relationship between pregnancy and the rate of postpartum hemorrhage. Cureus. 2022;**14**(6):e26460-e26467. Art. no. 6. DOI: 10.7759/cureus.26460

[82] Global Neonatal and Sepsis Initiative. The Global maternal and neonatal sepsis initiative: WHO. WHO: Sexual and reproductive health and rights - Global Maternal & Neonatal Sepsis Initiative. Available from: https://srhr.org/sepsis/ [Accessed: June 24, 2024]

[83] Pan American Health Organization (PAHO). Obstetric infections are the third most common cause of maternal mortality. Available from: https://www.paho.org/en/news/21-9-2020-obstetric-infections-are-third-most-common-cause-maternal-mortality-according-who [Accessed: June 24, 2024]

[84] The World Health Organization (WHO), Global Maternal Sepsis Study (GLOSS) Research Group, et al. Frequency and management of maternal infection in health facilities in 52 countries (GLOSS): A 1-week inception cohort study. The Lancet Global Health. 2020;**8**(5):e661-e671. Art. no. 5. DOI: 10.1016/S2214-109X(20)30109-1

[85] Global Neonatal and Sepsis Initiative. GLOSS, the global maternal sepsis study: World Health Organization. Global Maternal & Neonatal Sepsis Initiative. Available from: https://srhr.org/sepsis/gloss/ [Accessed: June 30, 2024]

[86] Jhpiego Corporation. Jhpiego: History & Mission. Jhpiego. Available from: https://www.jhpiego.org/about/history-mission/ [Accessed: June 24, 2024]

[87] Unger T et al. 2020 International Society of Hypertension Global Hypertension Practice Guidelines. Hypertension. 2020;**75**(6):1334-1357. Art. no. 6. DOI: 10.1161/hypertensionaha.120.15026

[88] Wang W et al. Epidemiological trends of maternal hypertensive disorders of pregnancy at the global, regional, and national levels: A population-based study. BMC Pregnancy and Childbirth. 2021;**21**(1):364-374. Art. no. 1. DOI: 10.1186/s12884-021-03809-2

[89] Miller EC, Vollbracht S. Neurology of preeclampsia and related disorders: An update in neuro-obstetrics. Current Pain and Headache Reports. 2021;**25**(6):40-61. Art. no. 6. DOI: 10.1007/s11916-021-00958-z

[90] Lathrop E, Jamieson DJ, Danel I. HIV and maternal mortality. International Journal of Gynecology & Obstetrics. 2014;**127**(2):213-215. Art. no. 2. DOI: 10.1016/j.ijgo.2014.05.024

[91] Calvert C, Ronsmans C. The contribution of HIV to pregnancy-related mortality: A systematic review and meta-analysis. AIDS (London, England). 2013;**27**(10):1631-1639. Art. no. 10. DOI: 10.1097/QAD.0b013e32835fd940

[92] Ssentongo P et al. Associations of malaria, HIV, and coinfection, with anemia in pregnancy in sub-Saharan Africa: A population-based cross-sectional study. BMC Pregnancy and Childbirth. 2020;**20**(1):379-390. Art. no. 1. DOI: 10.1186/s12884-020-03064-x

[93] The World Health Organization (WHO). Strategies to prevent anaemia: Recommendations from an expert group consultation, New Delhi, India, 5-6 December 2016. 2016. Available from: https://iris.who.int/handle/10665/312109 [Accessed: July 1, 2024]

[94] The World Health Organization (WHO). Nutritional Anaemias: Tools for Effective Prevention and Control. Geneva: World Health Organization; 2017. Available from: https://iris.who.int/handle/10665/259425 [Accessed: June 6, 2024]

[95] Steketee RW, Nahlen BL, Parise ME, Menendez C. The burden of malaria in pregnancy in malaria-endemic areas. In: The Intolerable Burden of Malaria: A New Look at the Numbers: Supplement to Volume 64(1) of the American Journal of Tropical Medicine and Hygiene, American Society of Tropical Medicine and Hygiene. 2001. Available from: https://www.ncbi.nlm.nih.gov/books/NBK2623/ [Accessed: July 1, 2024]

[96] Mansukhani R et al. Maternal anaemia and the risk of postpartum haemorrhage: A cohort analysis of data from the WOMAN-2 trial. The Lancet Global Health. 2023;**11**(8):e1249-e1259. Art. no. 8. DOI: 10.1016/S2214-109X(23)00245-0

[97] The United States Agency for International Development (USAID). Role of nutrition in preventing child and maternal deaths: Technical guidance brief on global health. USAID. Available from: https://www.usaid.gov/role-nutrition-preventing-child-and-maternal-deaths-technical-guidance-brief [Accessed: June 7, 2024]

[98] Saito M et al. Severe falciparum malaria in pregnancy in Southeast Asia: A multi-Centre retrospective cohort study. BMC Medicine. 2023;**21**(1):320-334. Art. no. 1. DOI: 10.1186/s12916-023-02991-8

[99] Brabin BJ, Hakimi M, Pelletier D. An analysis of anemia and pregnancy-related maternal mortality. The Journal of Nutrition. 2001;**131**(2):604S-615S. Art. no. 2. DOI: 10.1093/jn/131.2.604S

[100] The United Nations Population Fund (UNFPA), Rich mother, poor mother: The social determinants of maternal death and disability. 2012. Available from: https://www.unfpa.org/sites/default/files/resource-pdf/EN-SRH%20fact%20sheet-Poormother.pdf [Accessed: July 18, 2024]

[101] Greenberg MB, Gandhi M, Davidson C, Carter EB. Society for maternal-fetal medicine consult series #62: Best practices in equitable care delivery–addressing systemic racism and other social determinants of health as causes of obstetrical disparities. American Journal of Obstetrics and Gynecology. 2022;**227**(2):B44-B59. Art. no. 2. DOI: 10.1016/j.ajog.2022.04.001

[102] Minehart RD, Bryant AS, Jackson J, Daly JL. Racial/ethnic inequities in pregnancy-related morbidity and mortality. Obstetrics and Gynecology Clinics of North America. 2021;**48**(1):31-51. Art. no. 1. DOI: 10.1016/j.ogc.2020.11.005

[103] Slaughter-Acey J et al. Social and structural determinants of maternal morbidity and mortality: An evidence map. In: AHRQ Comparative Effectiveness Reviews. Rockville (MD): Agency for Healthcare Research and Quality (US); 2023. Available from: http://www.ncbi.nlm.nih.gov/books/NBK598895/

[104] The Centers for Disease Control and Prevention (CDC). Working together to reduce black maternal mortality | health equity features. Available from: https://www.cdc.gov/healthequity/features/maternal-mortality/index.html [Accessed: May 28, 2024]

[105] Rossen LM, Hoyert D, Branum AM. US trends in maternal mortality by racial and ethnic group. JAMA. 2023;**330**(18):1799-1800. DOI: 10.1001/jama.2023.17547

[106] Shlafer R, Saunders JB, Boraas CM, Kozhimannil KB, Mazumder N, Freese R. Maternal and neonatal outcomes among incarcerated women who gave birth

in custody. Birth Berkeley Calif. 2021;**48**(1):122-131. Art. no. 1. DOI: 10.1111/birt.12524

[107] Keygnaert I, Ivanova O, Guieu A, Parys A-SV, Leye E, Roelens K. Evidence on poor migrant maternal health. In: What Is the Evidence on the Reduction of Inequalities in Accessibility and Quality of Maternal Health Care Delivery for Migrants? A Review of the Existing Evidence in the WHO European Region [Internet]. WHO Regional Office for Europe; 2016. Available from: https://www.ncbi.nlm.nih.gov/books/NBK390813/ [Accessed: June 28, 2024]

[108] Pratt A, Fowler T. Deconstructing bias: Marginalization. 2022. Available from: https://science.nichd.nih.gov/confluence/pages/viewpage.action?pageId=242975243#:~:text=Today%2C%20the%20term%20marginalize%20is,considered%20%E2%80%9Cother%E2%80%9D%20within%20society [Accessed: July 18, 2024]

[109] Eslier M, Azria E, Chatzistergiou K, Stewart Z, Dechartres A, Deneux-Tharaux C. Association between migration and severe maternal outcomes in high-income countries: Systematic review and meta-analysis. PLoS Medicine. 2023;**20**(6):e1004257-e1004278. Art. no. 6. DOI: 10.1371/journal.pmed.1004257

[110] Kozhimannil KB, Interrante JD, Tofte AN, Admon LK. Severe maternal morbidity and mortality among indigenous women in the United States. Obstetrics and Gynecology. 2020;**135**(2):294-300. Art. no. 2. DOI: 10.1097/AOG.0000000000003647

[111] Lister RL, Drake W, BH S, Graves C. Black maternal mortality-the elephant in the room. World Journal of Gynecology & Womens Health. 2019;**3**(1):1-5. Art. no. 1

[112] National Institutes of Health (NIH). What factors increase the risk of maternal morbidity and mortality? Available from: https://www.nichd.nih.gov/health/topics/maternal-morbidity-mortality/conditioninfo/factors [Accessed: June 21, 2024]

[113] National Institutes of Health (NIH). Systemic racism, a key risk factor for maternal death and illness. Available from: https://www.nhlbi.nih.gov/news/2021/systemic-racism-key-risk-factor-maternal-death-and-illness [Accessed: July 7, 2024]

[114] Evans MK, Rosenbaum L, Malina D, Morrissey S, Rubin EJ. Diagnosing and treating systemic racism. The New England Journal of Medicine. 2020;**383**(3):274-276. DOI: 10.1056/NEJMe2021693

[115] National Institutes of Health (NIH). NIH study suggests women with disabilities have higher risk of birth complications and death. Available from: https://www.nih.gov/news-events/news-releases/nih-study-suggests-women-disabilities-have-higher-risk-birth-complications-death [Accessed: June 21, 2024]

[116] Gleason JL, Grewal J, Chen Z, Cernich AN, Grantz KL. Risk of adverse maternal outcomes in pregnant women with disabilities. JAMA Network Open. 2021;**4**(12):e2138414-e2138426. Art. no. 12. DOI: 10.1001/jamanetworkopen.2021.38414

[117] The World Health Organization (WHO). Adolescent pregnancy. Available from: https://www.who.int/news-room/fact-sheets/detail/adolescent-pregnancy [Accessed: June 21, 2024]

[118] National Institutes of Health (NIH). What are some factors that make a pregnancy high-risk? Available from:

https://www.nichd.nih.gov/health/topics/high-risk/conditioninfo/factors [Accessed: June 21, 2024]

[119] Kortekaas JC et al. Risk of adverse pregnancy outcomes of late- and post-term pregnancies in advanced maternal age: A national cohort study. Acta Obstetricia et Gynecologica Scandinavica. 2020;**99**(8):1022-1030. Art. no. 8. DOI: 10.1111/aogs.13828

[120] Ariel F, Asma H, Khadija M, Thea L. Maternal health and mortality—The story behind the numbers. Rabin Martin. Available from: https://rabinmartin.com/insights/maternal-health-and-mortality/. [Accessed: May 29, 2024]

[121] Moyo E, Dzinamarira T, Moyo P, Murewanhema G, Ross A. Men's involvement in maternal health in sub-Saharan Africa: A scoping review of enablers and barriers. Midwifery. 2024;**133**:103993. DOI: 10.1016/j.midw.2024.103993

[122] Gebretsadik LA, Mamo A, Koricha ZB, Morankar S. Effectiveness of targeted social and behavior change communication on maternal health knowledge, attitudes, and institutional childbirth: A cluster-randomized trial in Jimma zone, Ethiopia. European Journal of Public Health. 6 Jan 2025:ckae220. DOI: 10.1093/eurpub/ckae220

[123] Mirza MS, MSDW N, Monica C. Analysis of strategies for reducing maternal mortality rates (MMR) in developing countries: A meta-analysis. Sriwijaya Journal of Obstetrics and Gynecology. 2024;**2**(1):127-136. Art. no. 1. DOI: 10.59345/sjog.v2i1.140

[124] Kim J, Heazell AEP, Whittaker M, Stacey T, Watson K. Impact of health literacy on pregnancy outcomes in socioeconomically disadvantaged and ethnic minority populations: A scoping review. International Journal of Gynecology & Obstetrics. 2025;**168**(1):69-81. DOI: 10.1002/ijgo.15852

[125] Alvarado G, Schultz D, Malika N, Reed N. United States doula programs and their outcomes: A scoping review to inform state-level policies. Womens Health Issues. 2024;**34**(4):350-360. DOI: 10.1016/j.whi.2024.03.001

[126] Grunebaum A, Dudenhausen J, Chervenak FA. A crisis in U.S. maternal healthcare: Lessons from Europe for the U.S. Journal of Perinatal Medicine. 2025. DOI: 10.1515/jpm-2024-0606

[127] Sen A. Why health equity? Health Economics. 2002;**11**(8):659-666. DOI: 10.1002/hec.762

[128] Khosla R, Venkatapuram S. What is a justice-oriented approach to global health? BMJ Global Health. 2023;**8**(3):e012155. DOI: 10.1136/bmjgh-2023-012155

[129] Ahinkorah BO et al. Determinants of antenatal care and skilled birth attendance services utilization among childbearing women in Guinea: Evidence from the 2018 Guinea demographic and health survey data. BMC Pregnancy and Childbirth. 2021;**21**(1):2-13. Art. no. 1. DOI: 10.1186/s12884-020-03489-4

[130] Chilot D et al. Pooled prevalence and determinants of antenatal care visits in countries with high maternal mortality: A multi-country analysis. Frontiers in Public Health. 2023;**11**:1035759. DOI: 10.3389/fpubh.2023.1035759

Chapter 2

Cultural Influences on Labor and Delivery Practices

Bernadether Terentius Rugumisa

Abstract

Childbirth practices are deeply rooted in cultural traditions. These traditions encompass a wide range of beliefs, rituals, and societal norms that shape the experiences and decisions of women during pregnancy, labor, and delivery. Cultural influences include spiritual ceremonies, traditional knowledge, and practices passed down through generations. Modern medical interventions often coexist with or challenge traditional methods. Understanding and integrating these cultural dynamics into maternal care is essential for providing respectful, effective, and culturally sensitive healthcare. This chapter explores the historical and contemporary practices of childbirth across various cultures, highlighting the significant role of traditional birth attendants and the complex integration of modern medical practices. Additionally, it discusses the challenges in delivering culturally competent care. Through detailed case studies from different regions, the chapter emphasizes the importance of collaboration between healthcare providers and traditional practitioners. It also underscores the critical need for cultural competence training and the potential of technology to bridge communication gaps. The discussion suggests that a culturally sensitive approach to maternal care not only enhances the health outcomes for mothers and newborns but also promotes a more inclusive and equitable healthcare system that respects and values cultural diversity.

Keywords: cultural beliefs, traditional birth practices, healthcare integration, childbirth, birth rituals, traditional midwives, maternal health

1. Introduction

Culture profoundly shapes every aspect of human life, and childbirth is no exception. Cultural influences on labor and delivery practices include a broad spectrum of societal attitudes, beliefs, and religious traditions that collectively shape how childbirth is perceived and managed. These cultural elements influence the choices women make during pregnancy, the methods used during labor, and the acceptance or rejection of medical interventions [1]. Understanding these cultural dynamics is essential for healthcare providers to offer respectful, effective, and culturally sensitive care.

Societal attitudes toward childbirth vary significantly across different cultures. They impact access to care, the perceived role of medical intervention, and the support structures available to expectant mothers. Cultural beliefs, which include traditional knowledge and practices passed down through generations, play a crucial role in shaping childbirth experiences. These beliefs often dictate the use of specific rituals, customs, and pain management techniques during labor. Religious influences further add a layer of complexity, guiding practices and decisions with spiritual significance.

In many parts of the world, traditional childbirth practices remain integral to the cultural fabric of communities. These practices, while deeply rooted in tradition, often coexist with modern medical care. The integration of traditional and modern practices can present both challenges and opportunities, requiring a delicate balance to ensure that cultural values are respected while providing safe and effective medical care.

2. Historical context of childbirth

Throughout history, childbirth has been a deeply cultural experience influenced by the beliefs and practices of the community. Traditional birth practices have varied widely across different cultures and historical periods. In many societies, childbirth was primarily managed by women, with midwives and traditional birth attendants (TBAs) playing crucial roles. There are numerous examples from historic and cultural traditions that illustrate the deep intertwining of cultural beliefs and childbirth practices. We will journey through a few examples to explore the specific traditions surrounding childbirth, revealing how different cultures understood and celebrated the miracle of birth. Each tradition uniquely blended rituals, beliefs, and practices that have left a lasting impact on the way societies have approached the birthing process throughout history.

2.1 Ancient practices

In ancient Egypt, childbirth was considered a natural process that took place at home, often assisted by midwives who used herbal remedies and rituals to aid the delivery process and ensure the safety of both mother and child [2]. Women typically gave birth in a squatting position supported by birthing stools or bricks. The goddess Taweret, depicted as a pregnant hippopotamus, was regarded as a protector of women and children during childbirth. Taweret's image combined features of a hippopotamus, crocodile, and lioness—animals symbolizing strength and protection (**Figure 1**). Her association with childbirth extended beyond her form, as she was believed to ward off evil spirits and ensure the safe delivery [3]. Amulets and charms bearing Taweret's likeness were commonly used by expectant mothers, emphasizing her importance in Egyptian society as a symbol of fertility, maternity, and family protection.

Similarly, in ancient Greece, childbirth was overseen by goddesses like Eileithyia, the goddess of labor and childbirth [4]. Eileithyia was believed to have the power to either prolong or ease labor, making her presence crucial during the birthing process. Moreover, women believed the upright position helped with the delivery and they often used birth chairs to facilitate labor. Midwives played a crucial role of providing support and care to ease labor and had vast knowledge in using various herbs and techniques to assist with childbirth. Rituals and prayers served as significant practices during the childbirth process. Offerings were made to Eileithyia to seek her favor and intervention. In some places, small shrines were dedicated to her, where women could pray for a safe delivery. The goddess's influence was so profound that the city of Eileithyia in Crete was named after her, highlighting her importance in Greek culture and society.

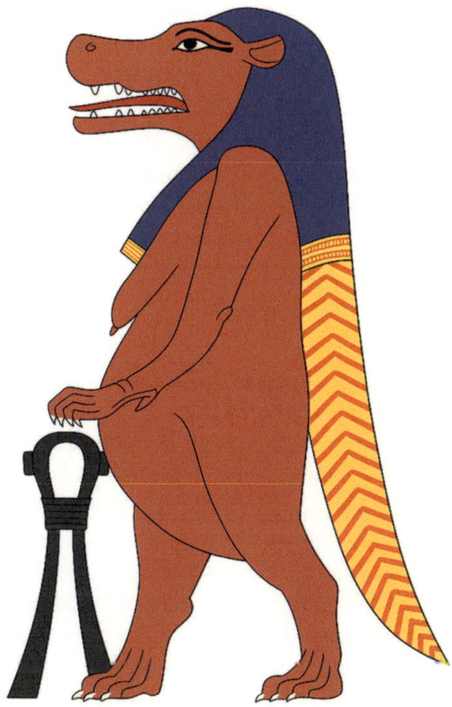

Figure 1.
Taweret, Egyptian goddess of fertility, motherhood, and childbirth (Image by Eternal Space, *licensed under Creative Commons Attribution-Share Alike 4.0 International (CC BY-SA 4.0). Source: Wikimedia Commons).*

In ancient China, childbirth was guided by the principles of traditional Chinese medicine (TCM) [5]. TCM emphasizes balance and harmony within the body. The goal of TCM was to ensure a smooth delivery by maintaining the equilibrium of yin and yang, as well as the flow of qi (life energy) through the body. Practices included the use of acupuncture to alleviate pain and stimulate labor by targeting specific points on the body. Also, the use of herbal remedies tailored to support the mother's health and promote the baby's safe passage. Specific dietary recommendations were also given to nourish the mother and strengthen her body during pregnancy and after childbirth. Midwives used the knowledge of TCM to manage pain and facilitate delivery, often employing techniques such as massage and moxibustion to encourage contractions and ease discomfort. These practices were deeply rooted in the philosophy of balance and natural processes, stressing the holistic approach to childbirth in ancient China. They demonstrated a deep understanding of the body's needs during this crucial period.

2.2 Indigenous practices

Among indigenous cultures in North America, childbirth was typically a communal and sacred event that was deeply integrated into the spiritual and social fabric of the community [6]. Native American tribes had specific rituals and practices designed to support the mother and ensure the well-being of the newborn. These rituals often involved prayers, songs, and the use of sacred objects to invoke the protection and guidance of ancestral spirits. Childbirth was seen as a natural aspect of life, and the entire community, including family members and spiritual leaders, often participated in or supported the event. Midwives and elder women assisted in the delivery, providing both physical and emotional support. They used herbal medicines and traditional techniques to manage pain and facilitate labor. The elder women were respected as keepers of wisdom, understanding the intricate balance between the physical and spiritual realms during childbirth. The birth of a child was celebrated as a continuation of the tribe's lineage and a reaffirmation of cultural identity.

2.3 Medieval and renaissance Europe

During the medieval period in Europe, childbirth took place at home and was managed primarily by midwives, who were the key figures in the birthing process. They used a range of traditional practices, including herbal remedies to ease pain and prevent infection, as well as massages to help relax the mother and encourage labor. Midwives also provided emotional support and comfort, creating a familiar and supportive environment for the birthing mother.

As medical knowledge progressed, the role of midwives began to decline with the rise of male-dominated medical professions. Physicians gained prominence, and they began to view childbirth as a medical procedure rather than a natural process. This led to a gradual shift toward more medicalized approaches to childbirth. The change was further driven by advancements in medical knowledge and the development of new surgical techniques.

The Renaissance period marked a significant increase in understanding of anatomy and the human body, contributing to the shift from home births to hospital deliveries [7]. Although the transition was slow, and many women continued to give birth at home, the perception of childbirth was gradually changing. The increasing involvement of male physicians in the birthing process reflected broader societal changes. There was a growing influence of science and medicine over traditional practices. This period laid the groundwork for the modern medicalized approach to childbirth that emerged in the centuries that followed.

2.4 Transition to modern obstetrics

The 18th and 19th centuries marked significant changes in childbirth practices, particularly in Western societies. The development of modern obstetrics introduced new medical interventions [7]. For instance, the use of forceps that allowed physicians to assist in difficult deliveries, thereby reducing infant mortality rates. The introduction of anesthesia in the form of ether and chloroform in the mid-nineteenth century revolutionized the birthing process by providing pain relief during labor, making childbirth a less traumatic experience for many women.

Pioneers like William Smellie and Ignaz Semmelweis made critical contributions to improving maternal and neonatal health [8]. William Smellie, a Scottish obstetrician, was instrumental in advancing the understanding of fetal anatomy and developing techniques to safely deliver babies. This contribution earned him recognition as a founding figure in modern obstetrics. Ignaz Semmelweis, a Hungarian physician, demonstrated the importance of hygiene in preventing infections during childbirth

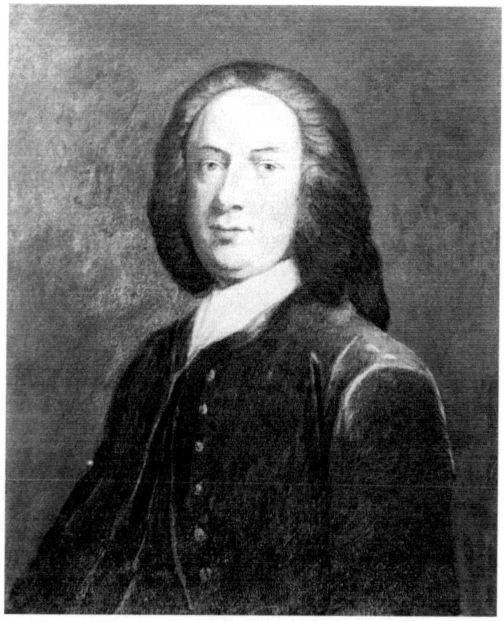

Figure 2.
Portrait of William Smellie. From the original painting in the Royal College of Surgeons, Edinburgh (Image credit: Wellcome Collection. Licensed under Creative Commons Attribution 4.0 International (CC BY 4.0). Source: Wellcome Collection).

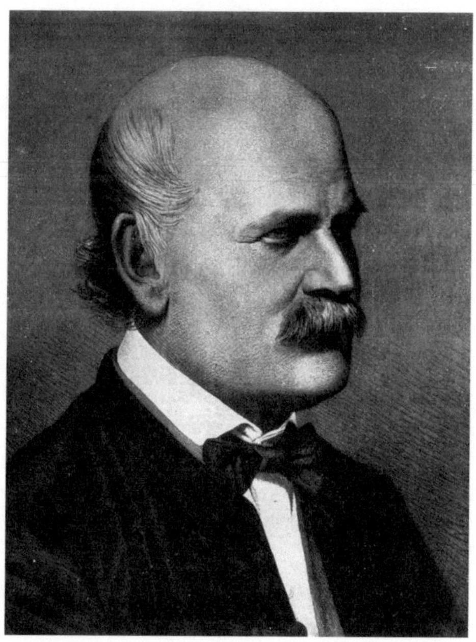

Figure 3.
Portrait of Ignaz Semmelweis (1858), a pioneering Hungarian physician known for his early advocacy of antiseptic procedures (This image is in the public domain. Source: Wikimedia Commons. Available at: Ignaz Semmelweis Portrait).

by introducing handwashing practices with chlorinated lime solutions in the mid-nineteenth century (**Figure 2**).

During this period, there was a gradual shift from home births attended by midwives to hospital births managed by physicians. This transition was influenced by the growing trust in medical science. People started to believe that hospitals provided safer environments due to their access to medical equipment and trained professionals. While the medical advancements improved maternal and neonatal outcomes, and reduces mortality rates, they also led to a diminished role of traditional birth attendants. The increased medicalization of childbirth marginalized midwives and traditional practices. Nonetheless, the shift toward clinical approaches occasionally overlooked the holistic and personal aspects of the birthing experience (**Figure 3**).

3. Contemporary practices and revival of traditional methods

Despite the dominance of modern medical practices, there is a growing interest in reviving traditional childbirth methods and blending them with contemporary techniques [9]. This move aims to honor and preserve cultural traditions while taking advantage of modern medical technology to improve maternal and neonatal health outcomes.

Natural childbirth methods, such as water births and the use of doulas, are gaining popularity in Western countries. Doulas are trained nonmedical professionals who provide continuous physical, emotional, and informational support before, during and shortly after delivery. They help mothers and their families achieve the healthiest and most satisfying birthing experience possible. In the United States, the inclusion of doulas in modern maternity care has led to improved maternal and neonatal outcomes [10].

In some African, countries like Ethiopia and Tanzania, community health workers train traditional birth attendants and midwives in areas with limited access to medical facilities [11]. They focus on teaching hygiene, recognizing signs of danger, and knowing when to refer a mother to healthcare facilities. In New Zealand, midwives are given professional training that allows them to collaborate with obstetricians to provide comprehensive care during pregnancy and childbirth. In Guatemala, traditional Mayan midwives, known as comadronas, work together with healthcare professionals to ensure safe deliveries while maintaining cultural practices [12]. Additionally, the Netherlands highly supports home births and has a well-established system that minimizes unnecessary medical interventions [13]. This approach is rooted in Dutch cultural beliefs about the naturalness of childbirth. However, in Brazil, cultural preferences and medical practices have led to a high rate of cesarean sections. Many people perceive cesarean deliveries as more convenient and safer [14].

4. Cultural, spiritual, and religious influences on childbirth

Childbirth is not only a biological event but also a deeply cultural, spiritual, and religious experience that reflects the values, beliefs, and practices of a community. Across the globe, the act of bringing new life into the world is surrounded by rich traditions, rituals, and communal practices that are integral to the cultural fabric of societies. These practices often intertwine spiritual beliefs with practical approaches to childbirth, ensuring that both the physical and spiritual well-being of the mother and child are safeguarded. In this section, we explore the role of family and community, rituals and traditions, and the spiritual and religious practices that influence childbirth across different cultures.

4.1 Role of family and community

In many cultures, childbirth is viewed not just as a personal or family event but as a communal affair that involves the entire community. The involvement of family members, friends, and even neighbors is often seen as essential to ensuring a safe and successful birth. While reinforcing social bonds and cultural legacy, the communal approach to childbirth emphasizes the collective responsibility for the well-being of the mother and child.

In Latin American cultures for example, the postpartum tradition known as *cuarentena* involves a period of approximately 40 days during which the mother is expected to rest and recuperate [15]. This period is marked by a strong support system, where female relatives and community members take on household chores and care for other children, allowing the mother to focus on bonding with her newborn. This tradition highlights the cultural importance placed on family and community support during the postpartum period. It reflects a deep understanding of the physical and emotional needs of the mother.

Similarly, in many African communities, childbirth is a time when women come together to offer support to the laboring mother. It is common for female relatives, friends, and neighbors to gather, offering encouragement and practical help throughout the labor and delivery process. This support network is not only crucial for the mother's well-being, but also serves to pass down traditional knowledge and practices related to childbirth. Elder women, in particular, hold respected positions, acting as custodians of wisdom and guiding younger women through the birthing process. Their involvement ensures the maintenance of cultural practices and reinforces community bonds.

The role of family and community in childbirth reflects the cultural belief that the arrival of a new life is a collective experience that strengthens familial ties and reaffirms social bonds. By embracing this approach, cultures not only ensure the physical wellbeing of the mother and child but also nurture the emotional and social aspects of childbirth, creating a supportive environment that benefits all involved.

4.2 Rituals and traditions

Rituals and traditions surrounding childbirth are integral to many cultures worldwide. These practices often embody deep spiritual, communal, and cultural significance. They go beyond the physical aspects of childbirth to encompass the emotional and spiritual dimensions of bringing new life into the world. Rituals are performed to protect the mother and newborn, honor the birth, and preserve cultural traditions.

Among Indigenous cultures, childbirth is often seen as a sacred event that is closely tied to the spiritual beliefs of the community. For example, in some Native American tribes, childbirth is accompanied by rituals designed to protect both the mother and the newborn. These rituals might include the use of sacred objects, prayers, and songs that invoke the protection and guidance of ancestral spirits. Elders and spiritual leaders often play a central role in these practices. They conduct ceremonies that connect the newborn to the spirits that will bless and protect babies as they enter the world. Such traditions highlight the importance of maintaining spiritual harmony and honoring the connections between past, present, and future generations.

In traditional Chinese culture, the postpartum period, known as "sitting the month" or *zuo yuezi*, involves a series of practices aiming at restoring the mother's health and ensuring the well-being of the baby [16]. During this time, the mother is cared for by family members and follows a special diet. The diet is believed to replenish energy and promote healing. The practice of *zuo yuezi* underscores a deep cultural understanding of the importance of postpartum care, and it emphasizes the role of family in nurturing the new mother and child. The cultural value placed on maternal health regards this period of rest and recovery as crucial for the long-term health of both the mother and the baby.

Generally, rituals and traditions play a critical role in shaping the childbirth experience. They offer both spiritual and practical support to the mother. These practices are deeply rooted in cultural beliefs and are often passed down through generations to ensure the continuity of cultural identity and the preservation of traditional knowledge.

4.3 Spiritual and religious practices

Religion and spirituality are deeply intertwined with culture and play a vital role in many people's lives. They influence numerous aspects, including childbirth, across different societies. Religious beliefs imbue the birthing process with profound spiritual significance by serving as a conduit for divine protection and guidance for both the mother and the newborn. The specifics of these practices vary widely across religions. However, they consistently highlight the intersection of faith, culture, and tradition and offer valuable insights into how different communities experience the miracle of birth.

In Islam, childbirth is a moment enriched with spiritual meaning and community celebration. One of the first rites of passage for a newborn Muslim is the recitation of the *Adhan* (call to prayer) into the baby's ear. This act symbolizes the child's formal entry into the Islamic faith and serves as a lifelong spiritual compass. Following this, the *Tahnik* ritual is performed, where a softened piece of date is placed in the baby's mouth, emulating the practices of the Prophet Muhammad. This ritual seeks blessings for the child's health and longevity. The Islamic tradition further celebrates the birth through the *Aqiqah* ceremony, which involves the sacrifice of an animal. The meat is distributed among family, friends, and the needy, symbolizing gratitude and fostering community support. Many Muslim women prefer to have a trusted female relative or midwife present during labor and delivery to maintain modesty.

Christianity also infuses the childbirth experience with spiritual rituals and blessings. For many Christian families, the presence of clergy, who offer prayers for safe delivery during childbirth, is a source of comfort and spiritual support. In some Christian traditions, special services or blessings are performed before or after childbirth to celebrate the new life. One of the most significant rites following birth is baptism, marking the child's entry into the Christian community. This ritual is a powerful symbol of purification and protection, seeking God's guidance and grace for the child's future. Some Christian denominations emphasize natural childbirth, viewing it as part of God's design for women. In some cases, the observance of the religious holidays can influence the timing and type of medical care sought.

In Buddhism, the core value of the faith in childbirth is approached with mindfulness and tranquility. Expectant mothers and their families engage in chanting and meditation to cultivate a serene and peaceful atmosphere during labor. These practices ensure harmonious environment for the birth by alleviating stress and promoting positive energy (**Figure 4**).

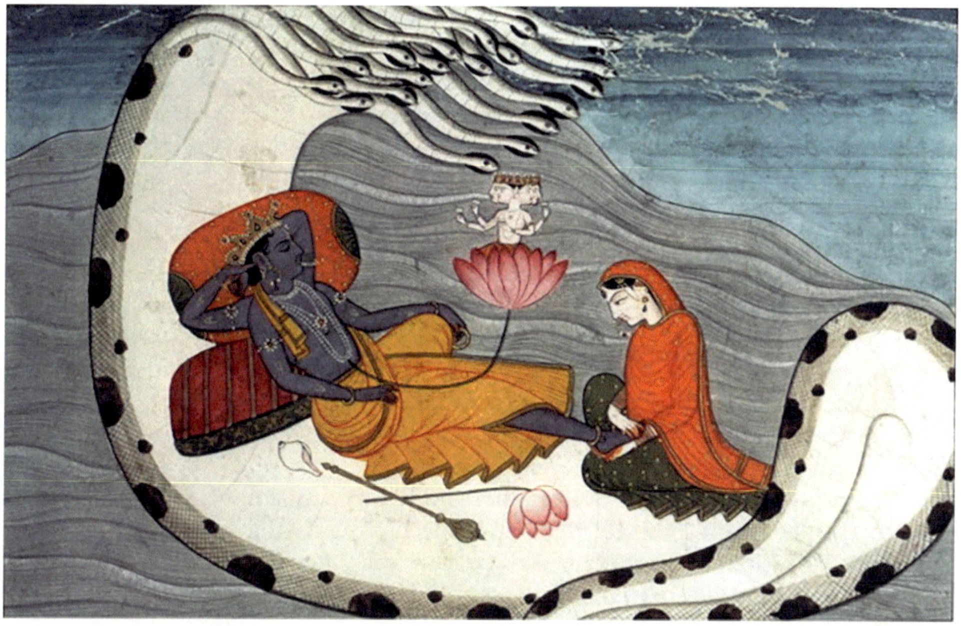

Figure 4.
Vishnu and Lakshmi on Shesha Naga, circa 1870 (This image is in the public domain. Courtesy of Wikimedia Commons. Available at: Vishnu and Lakshmi on Shesha Naga, ca 1870).

In Hindu culture, childbirth is considered a sacred event with divine significance, closely associated with the blessings of various deities. During pregnancy, rituals such as *Pumsavana* and *Simantonnayana* are conducted to seek blessings for the unborn child and ensure a healthy delivery. These ceremonies often involve offerings, prayers, and the chanting of mantras dedicated to deities like Vishnu and Lakshmi, who are believed to protect the mother and child throughout the pregnancy.

Spiritual and religious practices surrounding childbirth serve as a means of seeking divine protection and blessings for the mother and newborn. These practices are deeply rooted in the religious beliefs of the community and are often accompanied by rituals that reinforce the spiritual significance of bringing new life into the world.

5. Pain management and coping strategies during labor

Pain management and coping strategies during labor are profoundly influenced by cultural, spiritual, and religious beliefs. Across the globe, diverse approaches are employed, ranging from medical interventions to traditional practices that incorporate spiritual and emotional support. These methods represent each culture's understanding of childbirth and its significance. They also offer unique perspectives on managing one of life's most challenging yet rewarding experiences.

5.1 Holistic and spiritual approaches

In India, for example, Ayurvedic practices offer a holistic approach to managing labor pain by emphasizing the interconnectedness of body, mind, and spirit [17]. These practices transform childbirth into a multidimensional experience, where the physical and emotional aspects are intricately linked. Expectant mothers are provided with herbal oils and massages, for the purpose of easing physical discomfort and promoting emotional well-being. The integration of breathing exercises and meditation further enhances this holistic approach, facilitating focus and serenity. Such techniques reflect the Ayurvedic philosophy that true wellness arises from the harmonious balance of all aspects of being. Through this, mothers are offered a comprehensive pathway to navigate the challenges of labor.

In many Indigenous cultures, spirituality is a cornerstone of childbirth, infusing the process with sacred significance. Within Native American communities, childbirth is revered as a profound spiritual journey. Rituals, such as smudging with sage, purify the environment, creating a space conducive to positive energy and spiritual support. The rhythmic sounds of chanting and drumming provide a soothing backdrop, reinforcing the connection between the laboring mother and her community. These practices draw on ancestral wisdom, offering spiritual tools for managing pain and promoting resilience during labor.

Both Ayurvedic and Indigenous practices underscore the importance of viewing pain management during childbirth as a holistic experience that transcends mere physical intervention. By embracing the spiritual and emotional dimensions of labor, these approaches provide a deeper understanding of how cultures integrate traditional knowledge and spiritual practices to support women in managing pain.

5.2 Traditional methods and modern interventions

In Western cultures, the clinical environment of hospitals offers a range of medical interventions for pain relief, such as epidural anesthesia and intravenous medications. However, there is a growing movement toward incorporating holistic methods like hypnobirthing, which combines relaxation and visualization techniques to help mothers manage pain naturally. This fusion of medical science and holistic practices exemplifies a broader trend of integrating traditional wisdom with modern advancements.

Similarly, TCM offers a harmonious blend of ancient and contemporary practices. Acupuncture and acupressure, rooted in thousands of years of tradition, are employed to stimulate energy flow and reduce pain during labor. These techniques reflect a deep understanding of the body's natural rhythms and emphasize a balanced approach to childbirth.

5.3 Community and cultural support

In African cultures, childbirth is a communal event where support from family and friends is integral to the birthing process. Women from the community, including elder relatives and friends, gather to provide encouragement, perform massages, and apply herbal remedies that help manage pain. This network of support fosters a sense of solidarity and ensures that the mother does not face the challenges of labor alone.

TBAs are often central to this community support system. They not only offer practical assistance during childbirth but also provide a deep connection to cultural traditions and spiritual practices. Their role is especially significant in rural and underserved areas, where access to modern medical facilities may be limited. However, the role of TBAs goes beyond just being part of the community support system. Their role in maternal care is extensive and will further be explored in the next section.

Across these varied approaches for pain management, a common thread emerges: the recognition of childbirth as a profound journey that encompasses physical, emotional, and spiritual dimensions. Whether through medical interventions, holistic practices, or spiritual rituals, the diverse strategies for managing pain during labor reflect the rich tapestry of human experience and the enduring importance of culture and tradition in shaping childbirth practices.

6. Role of traditional birth attendants

For centuries, in many communities worldwide, TBAs have been integral to maternal healthcare, particularly in rural and underserved areas [11]. These attendants are often respected members of the community, trusted for their knowledge of childbirth and their ability to provide compassionate care. They often serve as the primary caregivers during pregnancy, childbirth, and the postpartum period, providing culturally appropriate care and support to expectant mothers. Typically, TBAs acquire their skills through apprenticeships passed down through generations, making them deeply embedded in the cultural fabric of the communities they serve. In many African, Asian, and Latin American societies, TBAs are viewed as custodians of cultural birthing practices, which may include specific rituals, herbal remedies, and spiritual ceremonies. These practices are integral to the community's identity and are often valued alongside modern medical interventions.

In terms of maternal care, TBAs provide a range of services including physical care as well as emotional and spiritual support. TBAs monitor the pregnancy's progress, provide culturally relevant advice, and serve as a bridge between the mother and the healthcare system. During labor, TBAs offer hands-on assistance using traditional techniques to facilitate delivery. They provide comfort and reassurance in a supportive environment that respects cultural beliefs and practices. After childbirth, TBAs continue to support new mothers by offering advice on breastfeeding, newborn care, and recovery. Also, they offer prenatal care by guiding nutrition, hygiene, and prenatal exercises, helping expectant mothers prepare for childbirth. They may also perform traditional rituals that celebrate the new life and ensure the mother's well-being.

While TBAs are vital in many communities, integrating their practices with modern healthcare systems presents both challenges and opportunities. Among the key challenges is ensuring that TBAs receive adequate training and education to recognize and respond to complications that require medical intervention. Training programs can enhance their skills, improve maternal and infant outcomes, and strengthen collaboration between TBAs and healthcare professionals. TBAs can play a crucial role in increasing access to maternal healthcare services, particularly in remote areas. By working closely with healthcare providers, TBAs can help identify high-risk pregnancies and facilitate timely referrals to medical facilities, thereby bridging gaps in healthcare delivery.

Moreover, TBAs bring cultural sensitivity to maternal care, ensuring that cultural practices are respected and integrated into healthcare services. This can enhance patient satisfaction, trust in the healthcare system, and better health outcomes. However, in many low-resource settings, TBAs may have limited ability to provide safe and effective care due to lack of access to essential medical supplies and equipment. Addressing these resource constraints is critical for improving the quality of care TBAs can offer.

The role of TBAs is evolving as healthcare systems seek to integrate traditional practices with modern medical care. By acknowledging the value of TBAs and providing them with training and resources, healthcare systems can improve maternal and neonatal health outcomes while respecting cultural practices. Initiatives to support TBAs include training programs focused on recognizing complications, providing safe delivery techniques, and educating on modern healthcare practices. These programs aim to empower TBAs by enhancing their role as key partners in maternal healthcare.

The collaboration between TBAs and healthcare providers offers a pathway to more inclusive and culturally sensitive healthcare systems. By valuing the unique contributions of TBAs, communities can create environments where maternal health is prioritized, leading to healthier families and stronger communities.

7. Societal attitudes, gender roles, and maternal health

The experiences of women during pregnancy, childbirth, and postpartum care are profoundly shaped by the societal attitudes and gender roles prevalent in their communities. These factors influence not only how women access and receive healthcare but also how they perceive their own health and well-being. Societal attitudes toward motherhood and childbirth vary widely across cultures. In some societies, motherhood is idealized and considered a central aspect of a woman's identity. While this can lead to strong social support systems, it can also place immense pressure on women to conform to traditional expectations.

In cultures where motherhood is highly valued, women may receive extensive support during pregnancy and childbirth, which can lead to positive health outcomes. However, these same attitudes can also result in stigmatization of women who face challenges, such as infertility, pregnancy complications, or those who choose not to have children. The societal expectation to conform to a maternal role can lead to psychological stress and reluctance to seek help when needed.

Societal attitudes also influence how readily women can access healthcare services. In some communities, traditional beliefs may lead to a preference for home births and the use of traditional birth attendants, while in others, there may be a strong reliance on medicalized childbirth in hospitals. Understanding these attitudes is essential for healthcare providers to offer appropriate, culturally sensitive care.

7.1 Gender roles and maternal health

Gender roles play a pivotal role in shaping women's experiences during pregnancy and childbirth. In many societies, traditional gender roles dictate that women are primarily responsible for childbearing and caregiving. Such roles can have both positive and negative implications for women's health.

In patriarchal societies, women may have limited autonomy over their healthcare decisions. Male family members or community leaders often make critical choices regarding where and how a woman gives birth. This system can delay access to necessary medical interventions and increase the risk of complications. Empowering women in these societies with the ability to make informed decisions about their own healthcare is crucial for improving maternal health outcomes.

Moreover, gender roles often reinforce economic dependence on male partners, which can restrict women's access to healthcare services. Women who lack financial independence may struggle to afford prenatal care, proper nutrition, or safe childbirth services. The economic dependency can also lead to delayed healthcare-seeking behavior, as women may prioritize the needs of the family over their own health.

7.2 Cultural stigmas and their impact on maternal health

Cultural stigmas related to pregnancy and childbirth can have severe consequences for maternal health. These stigmas often arise from deeply ingrained societal norms and gender roles, and they can prevent women from seeking the care they need. In cultures where pregnancy complications or issues such as infertility are stigmatized, affected women are likely to face social isolation and inadequate support. The stigma can cause women to delay seeking medical help, exacerbating health issues and leading to poorer outcomes for both the mother and the child.

Additionaly, women may feel pressured to endure labor pain without seeking relief due to cultural expectations that honor suffering or stoicism. In some societies, the use of pain relief during childbirth may be discouraged, as it is seen as weakening the mother or interfering with natural processes. This cultural pressure can result in women having traumatic birth experiences, which could have been mitigated with appropriate pain management.

7.3 Economic and political influences

Economic and political factors interact with cultural and gender attitudes to shape societal perspectives on maternal health. In economically prosperous societies, maternal health is often prioritized through well-funded healthcare systems that provide comprehensive services and support for expectant mothers. These systems are often influenced by cultural values that emphasize women's health and well-being, leading to better maternal health outcomes.

In contrast, in economically disadvantaged regions, limited resources and cultural norms that devalue women's health can hinder the development of effective maternal health programs. Political instability and lack of government commitment can further exacerbate these challenges, highlighting the need for culturally appropriate interventions that address these systemic issues.

Changing societal attitudes toward maternal health requires a concerted effort to respect and integrate cultural beliefs and gender roles while prioritizing the health and well-being of women and their families. Through education, advocacy, and culturally and gender-sensitive policies, societies can create environments that support maternal health and empower women, leading to healthier families and communities.

8. Challenges and opportunities in culturally sensitive maternal care

In the pursuit of improving maternal health outcomes worldwide, culturally sensitive care has emerged as a crucial component. Understanding and integrating cultural beliefs, practices, and social norms into healthcare delivery is essential for providing effective and respectful care. However, the path to achieving culturally sensitive maternal care is fraught with challenges. At the same time, these challenges present unique opportunities for innovation and improvement in healthcare delivery. This section explores the current challenges, the opportunities for progress, and the future directions for advancing culturally sensitive maternal care.

8.1 Challenges in culturally sensitive maternal care

One of the primary challenges in providing culturally sensitive care is the diversity of cultural beliefs and practices across different communities [18]. Healthcare providers must have a broad understanding of different cultural norms, values, and practices related to childbirth and maternal health. In many cases, healthcare providers may lack the training or resources needed to effectively understand and respect these cultural differences. This can lead to misunderstandings, miscommunication, and a lack of trust between patients and providers.

Language barriers also pose significant challenges in delivering culturally sensitive care. Effective communication is the cornerstone of quality healthcare. However, failure to understand each other often prevent healthcare providers from fully understanding their patients' needs or explaining medical procedures clearly. In maternal care, this can lead to misunderstandings about treatment options, consent, and the importance of follow-up care. Language barriers can also contribute to feelings of isolation and anxiety among expectant mothers, particularly if they cannot express their concerns or preferences.

Another challenge is the lack of widespread training in cultural competence for healthcare providers. Many healthcare professionals receive limited education on how to provide care that respects and integrates cultural beliefs and practices. Without this training, providers may inadvertently impose their own cultural values on patients, leading to a lack of trust and poor patient–provider relationships. The absence of culturally competent training can result in a disconnect between healthcare systems and the communities they serve.

Lastly, in many low-resource settings, healthcare systems are stretched thin with limited staff, supplies, and infrastructure. These constraints make it challenging to provide personalized, culturally sensitive care. Overburdened healthcare workers may not have the time or resources to engage in meaningful conversations about cultural practices or to accommodate traditional birthing practices. Additionally, systemic biases within healthcare institutions can further marginalize certain cultural groups, leading to disparities in maternal health outcomes.

8.2 Opportunities for advancing culturally sensitive care

Despite the challenges, there are significant opportunities to improve culturally sensitive care and enhance maternal health outcomes. One key opportunity is the development of training programs that focus on cultural competence for healthcare providers. These programs can educate providers about the cultural beliefs and practices of the communities they serve, improving their ability to offer respectful and effective care. Training can include practical skills, such as communicating across language barriers, recognizing cultural stigmas, and incorporating traditional practices into care plans. By fostering cultural competence, healthcare systems can build trust with diverse populations and improve maternal health outcomes.

Collaboration with community leaders and traditional birth attendants offers another opportunity to enhance culturally sensitive care. By working with individuals who are respected and trusted within their communities, healthcare providers can gain valuable insights into cultural practices and preferences. This collaboration can facilitate the integration of traditional practices with modern medical care, ensuring that cultural beliefs are respected while maintaining a focus on safety and efficacy.

Technology also offers innovative solutions to some of the challenges associated with culturally sensitive care. Translation apps, telehealth services, and culturally appropriate educational materials can help bridge communication gaps and ensure that patients understand their healthcare options. Mobile health (mHealth) platforms can also be used to deliver culturally tailored health information, empowering women with knowledge about their pregnancies and childbirth options [19]. These technologies can make culturally sensitive care more accessible, particularly in remote or underserved areas.

Finally, community engagement is key to developing culturally sensitive healthcare services. By involving community leaders, traditional healers, and local organizations in the design and delivery of maternal health programs, healthcare providers can ensure that services are culturally appropriate and responsive to community needs. Community-based interventions, such as health education workshops or support groups for expectant mothers, can foster a sense of trust and collaboration between healthcare providers and the communities they serve. These interventions also provide a platform for addressing cultural stigmas and promoting positive health behaviors.

9. Case studies of cultural influence on labor and delivery

Understanding the impact of cultural practices on labor and delivery through detailed case studies provides valuable insights into the diverse approaches to childbirth around the world.

In the remote Arctic regions of Canada, the Inuit have maintained traditional childbirth practices closely tied to their cultural heritage [20]. The creation of birthing centers in Inuit communities, such as the Rankin Inlet Birthing Centre, allows women to give birth closer to home while still having access to medical care if needed. These centers respect and incorporate Inuit cultural practices, improving maternal and neonatal outcomes by providing culturally appropriate care.

In Guatemala, traditional Mayan midwives, known as comadronas, play a crucial role in maternal healthcare, especially in rural areas [21]. Comadronas provide prenatal care, assist with deliveries, and offer postpartum support using a combination of traditional knowledge and practices. Training programs enhance their skills in recognizing complications and ensuring safe deliveries, significantly reducing maternal and neonatal mortality rates.

Among the Maasai people of Kenya and Tanzania, childbirth is a communal event supported by TBAs and elder women. Community health programs train TBAs in basic medical skills and emergency care, facilitating timely referrals to healthcare facilities [22]. This collaboration between TBAs and healthcare providers combines cultural practices with essential medical interventions, improving maternal health outcomes.

In the United Kingdom, the integration of water births into modern medical care offers a culturally sensitive option for women seeking a natural childbirth experience. Hospitals and birthing centers have adopted water births as a standard option, supported by trained midwives who ensure safety [23]. This initiative respects cultural preferences while providing necessary medical oversight, leading to positive outcomes for mothers and babies.

In the United States, the use of doulas has been integrated into modern maternity care. Programs like the Doula Project in New York City incorporate doulas into hospital settings, providing culturally competent care that respects the preferences and traditions of diverse communities. Research demonstrates that the presence of a doula during labor leads to shorter labor times, lower rates of cesarean sections, and higher satisfaction with the childbirth experience [10].

In Japan, birthing homes offer an alternative to hospital deliveries, blending traditional Japanese practices with modern medical care [24]. These facilities are staffed by midwives who provide a supportive environment for natural childbirth. Birthing homes emphasize minimal medical intervention, use of traditional pain relief methods, and incorporation of cultural practices. This model has gained popularity and is associated with high levels of maternal satisfaction and positive birth outcomes.

10. Conclusion

The journey toward enhancing maternal health care through culturally sensitive practices is both a complex and rewarding endeavor. As we have explored, integrating cultural competence into healthcare delivery is essential for meeting the diverse needs of expectant mothers worldwide. By acknowledging and respecting the cultural beliefs and practices that shape women's experiences of pregnancy and childbirth, healthcare providers can build trust, improve communication, and ultimately enhance health outcomes.

Collaboration is key in this effort. Partnering with community leaders and traditional birth attendants is essential for tailoring healthcare services to local customs and preferences. Such partnerships ensure that care is culturally relevant and accessible, building stronger relationships between healthcare systems and the communities they serve. Additionally, leveraging technology to bridge language barriers and extend access to care, especially in underserved areas, can significantly enhance the quality of maternal health services.

To achieve these goals, it is important to support community-based interventions and policy initiatives that prioritize culturally sensitive care. Empowering women through education and fostering environments that respect their healthcare decisions are key steps toward improving maternal health outcomes. Continued research and interdisciplinary collaboration will provide valuable insights for refining these strategies and ensuring they remain responsive to cultural dynamics.

Ultimately, creating a healthcare system that is inclusive and equitable is vital for delivering high-quality maternal care to all women, regardless of their cultural background. By embracing the rich cultural diversity and integrating it into healthcare practices, we can build a future where every mother and child receives the care they deserve, leading to healthier families and stronger communities. Through concerted efforts in training, collaboration, innovation, and empowerment, we can move toward a world where culturally sensitive care is not just an aspiration, but a reality for all.

Acknowledgements

I would like to thank Dr. Mary Suke for her encouragement to accept the invitation to contribute to this book. Her belief that passion can drive success was instrumental in my decision.

The author acknowledges the use of Elicit for literature review and ChatGPT OpenAI for enhancing workflow and language refinement.

Conflict of interest

The author declares no conflict of interest.

Author details

Bernadether Terentius Rugumisa
Mbeya University of Science and Technology, Mbeya, Tanzania

*Address all correspondence to: kokurugumisa@gmail.com

References

[1] Davis-Floyd RE. Birth as an American Rite of Passage. 2nd ed. Berkeley: University of California Press; 2004

[2] Wegner JW. Birthing in ancient Egypt. In: Wilkinson T, editor. The Egyptian World. London: Routledge; 2009. pp. 185-199

[3] Pinch G. Handbook of Egyptian Mythology. Santa Barbara: ABC-CLIO; 2002

[4] King H. Hippocrates' Woman: Reading the Female Body in Ancient Greece. London: Routledge; 1998

[5] Furth C. A Flourishing Yin: Gender in China's Medical History: 960-1665. Berkeley: University of California Press; 1999

[6] Miller JR, Ridington R. Native American Mythology. New York: Oxford University Press; 1997

[7] Porter R. The Greatest Benefit to Mankind: A Medical History of Humanity from Antiquity to the Present. London: HarperCollins; 1997

[8] Cunningham A. The Making of Modern Medicine: Science and Society in the Era of William Smellie and Ignaz Semmelweis. Cambridge: Cambridge University Press; 1990

[9] Cindoglu D, Sayan-Cengiz F. Medicalization discourse and modernity: Contested meanings over childbirth in contemporary Turkey. Health Care for Women International. 2010;**31**(3):221-243

[10] Kozhimannil KB, Hardeman RR, Attanasio LB, Blauer-Peterson C, O'Brien M. Doula care, birth outcomes, and costs among medicaid beneficiaries. American Journal of Public Health. 2015;**103**(4):e113-e121

[11] World Health Organization. WHO Recommendations on Health Promotion Interventions for Maternal and Newborn Health 2015. Geneva: World Health Organization; 2015

[12] Chaudhry S, Oliveira J, Shirazian T. The emerging role of the comadrona as a broker between ancient cultural beliefs and modern biomedicalization to improve maternal health care in Guatemala. In: Maternal Death and Pregnancy-Related Morbidity among Indigenous Women of Mexico and Central America: An Anthropological, Epidemiological, and Biomedical Approach. Cham, Switzerland: Springer International Publishing; 2018. pp. 599-616

[13] Wiegers TA. The quality of maternity care services as experienced by women in the Netherlands. BMC Pregnancy and Childbirth. 2009;**9**(1):1-10

[14] Freitas PF, Pereira CF, Urpia TS. Cesarean sections in Brazil: Demographic, socioeconomic, and cultural factors. Revista de Saúde Pública. 2019;**53**:52

[15] Piperata BA. Forty days and forty nights: A biocultural perspective on postpartum practices in the Amazon. Social Science and Medicine. 2008;**67**(7):1094-1103

[16] Raven JH, Chen Q, Tolhurst RJ, Garner P. Traditional beliefs and practices in the postpartum period in Fujian Province, China: A qualitative study. BMC Pregnancy and Childbirth. 2007;**7**:1-1

[17] Pitman V. The Nature of the Whole: Holism in Ancient Greek and Indian Medicine. Delhi: Motilal Banarsidass Publisher; 2006

[18] Truong M, Paradies Y, Priest N. Interventions to improve cultural competency in healthcare: A systematic review of reviews. BMC Health Services Research. 2014;**14**(1):99

[19] Lee SH, Nurmatov UB, Nwaru BI, Mukherjee M, Grant L, Pagliari C. Effectiveness of mHealth interventions for maternal, newborn and child health in low- and middle-income countries: Systematic review and meta-analysis. Journal of Global Health. 2016;**6**(1):010401

[20] Douglas V. Childbirth among the Canadian Inuit: A review of the clinical and cultural literature. International Journal of Circumpolar Health. 2006;**65**(2):117-132

[21] Juarez M, Austad K, Rohloff P. Lay midwives: On the front lines of the fight against maternal mortality in rural Guatemala. The American Journal of Tropical Medicine and Hygiene. 2019;**100**(2):237

[22] Warren C, Mwangi A, Oweya E, Kamunyu L, Koskei N. Strengthening community health worker programs through increased community engagement: Lessons from Kenya. BMC Health Services Research. 2020;**20**(1):1011

[23] Bates V, Crane J, Fannin M. Fluid modernities: The birthing pool in late twentieth-century Britain. Medical Humanities. 2024;**50**(2):312-321

[24] Behruzi R, Hatem M, Fraser W, Goulet L, Ii M, Misago C. Facilitators and barriers in the humanization of childbirth practice in Japan. BMC Pregnancy and Childbirth. 2010;**10**:1-8

Chapter 3

Intrapartum Care and Companionship during Labour and Delivery in a Low-Resource Setting

Unice Goshomi, Owen Goshomi and Angelline Goshomi

Abstract

Companionship is deemed critical in calming and making women cognisant of the physiology of labour and the associated coping mechanisms to be applied. Accordingly, companionship has the ability to mitigate the disturbing experience related to physical discomfort and severe pain inherent in the labour process. Companionship is about being with the woman physically, thus facilitating the tolerance of physical pain and emotional distress. While the practice of companionship is associated with physical presence and is highly acceptable as good practice worldwide, 'physical presence' has proved to be almost impossible to achieve in low-resource settings due to infrastructure challenges. This leaves room for identifying context-specific solutions while being mindful of not compromising the quality of care. Hence, the emergence of the concept of 'psychological presence' where the woman feels connected to their companions away from the bedside. This chapter aims to coin the concept of 'psychological presence' into companionship.

Keywords: physical presence, psychological presence, companionship, low-resource country, intrapartum care

1. Introduction

Labour pain is induced by uterine muscle contractions and cervical pressure from the presenting part. This pain may manifest as intense cramping in the belly, groin, and back, accompanied by a dull ache. Some women also experience soreness in their flanks or thighs [1–3]. Additional sources of discomfort during labour encompass pressure exerted on the bladder and bowels by the baby's head, as well as the distension of the birth canal as the baby progresses through it.

All resulting nerve transmissions (visceral and somatic) are transported to the dorsal horn neurons, where they are interpreted and conveyed to the brain through the spinothalamic tract [1–3]. The transmission to the hypothalamus and limbic systems facilitates the emotional and physiological responses linked to pain, like stress and anxiety. There is available evidence that the presence of continuous support from the woman's partner, close family members, or friends favours good labour progress.

 IntechOpen

Though there is no rule about who should accompany her, most importantly, it is about her choice; that is the one the mother wants as her birth companion. In labour, companionship will empower the pregnant woman to choose an individual of her choice who is willing and able to assume the position of a companion [2–4]. However, clear instructions to the companion are necessary to regulate the practices of companions and health professionals during labour companionship to prevent potential harm to the labouring mother.

1.1 Birth/labour companionship

1.1.1 Benefits of companionship

1.1.1.1 Social support

A labour companion of choice during childbirth is crucial for improving women's birth experience and confidence to give birth [4, 5]. Companionship has been linked with a number of benefits. The medical benefits of companionship have been recognised within medical and social care [6]. The positive effect of friendship on wound healing is evident in people with good social contacts who demonstrate faster wound repair than those in social isolation. The importance of genuine connections cannot be understated; for instance, having an active listener in one's life, combined with the joy of shared experiences, contributes to the overall enhancement of well-being. Emotional support in the form of constant presence, reassurance, and praise, as well as information about signs and symptoms of labour and the progress of labour, can be beneficial [5, 7].

Research has shown that individuals who lack social contact and those who do not participate in social activities have been shown to be at risk of developing chronic conditions. In a study conducted by Holopainen and Hakulinen [8], loneliness among people who lack quality friendships, romantic partnerships, or other relationships increases the risks of heart attack, stroke, and premature death.

A lack of companionship is not only associated with depressive symptoms but it has also been proven to have a significant effect on physical health. Social isolation has been linked to a variety of conditions, such as cardiovascular disease [5]. Companionship is therefore so necessary as it leads to a better enjoyment of life and improved well-being.

1.1.1.2 Psychological support

The benefits of friendship are psychological as well. The companionate function of friendship supports positive mental health and serves to support individuals during stressful life events. Loneliness has been found to be negatively correlated with happiness and perceived life satisfaction. Alcoholism, depression, psychosomatic illness, and poor self-esteem are also more common among lonely people [6]. Loneliness is also a factor in poor sleep patterns and could contribute to the progression of dementia. Living a life of solitude can also contribute to a shorter life expectancy [8]. In labour, a key component of achieving respectful maternal and newborn care is labour companionship. Despite important health benefits for the woman and baby, there are critical gaps in implementing labour companionship for all women globally [9].

Companionship can also help reduce stress by releasing endorphins, which are hormones that make you feel good. Friends and family provide a space for us to share our joys and sorrows, express our passions, and find comfort in trying times [10]. Inner well-being is also greatly impacted by companionship.

1.1.1.3 Emotional support

Emotional support has been identified as a central aspect of companionship, where companions provide reassurance, comfort, and empathy to the labouring woman. This form of support is often seen as essential in reducing anxiety and fostering a sense of security during the birthing process [4, 11, 12]. Companionship care provides a support system where burdens are shared and problems are solved together. Carers actively create opportunities for social engagement and community involvement. With this aim, our skilled carers play a pivotal role in preventing isolation [5]. Providing a positive perception to the mother to not regard labour as a painful process but rather as the process of giving birth to another human being. Supported by someone who is physically present. The continuous physical presence of a trusted person provides the mother with both emotional and practical support. This constant presence is associated with increased confidence and reduced feelings of isolation during labour [13].

1.1.1.4 Advocacy

It is argued that advocacy as a critical element of companionship, where the companion plays a role in ensuring the mother's preferences are communicated and respected by the medical team, empowers women by giving them a voice during labour and delivery [12, 14]. The author identified that companions often act as advocates for the mother, ensuring that her preferences and rights are respected during labour. This advocacy plays a crucial role in protecting the mother's autonomy and ensuring that medical decisions align with her wishes [4]. It has also been noted that advocacy in companionship includes aiding in communication between the mother and healthcare providers, facilitating better understanding and cooperation. This support helps ensure that the woman's needs and concerns are addressed promptly and effectively during labour [11, 15, 16]. Ultimately helping the labouring mothers in making sound decisions, helping the mother navigate medical choices, and advocating for informed consent. A process that assists mothers in feeling more in control and less overwhelmed by complex medical interventions [4]. Keeping the woman conversant about the progress of her labour is critical. The woman and her companion have the right to know what is happening to the progress of their labour and the condition and that of the baby. Counselling the woman and her companion is about continuing care, which includes physical care, comfort, and emotional support. Inform the woman and her support person early in labour, before it becomes too painful, on what to expect. They should be aware that the contractions will become stronger and closer together when labour progresses towards delivery [1, 2]. Reassure the woman and their support that you will also be available for them [1, 2].

1.1.1.5 Pain management

The authors highlighted that companions through physical touch and emotional reassurance help in managing labour pain. Techniques such as massages, verbal encouragement, and breathing exercises facilitated by companions contribute to reducing the perception of pain and the need for medical interventions [11, 15].

1.1.1.6 Improved maternal outcomes

According to Yaya et al. and Waterhouse and O'Connor [9, 10], companionship during labour is associated with improved maternal outcomes, such as reduced rates of caesarean sections, fewer interventions, and shorter labour durations. Companionship was linked with enhanced physiological and psychological well-being in mothers.

1.2 Sources of companionship in labour

1.2.1 Birth partner

A birth partner is often the spouse or a close family member, as a common form of companionship. Birth partners are integral in providing both emotional and physical support, reinforcing the mother's comfort and reducing feelings of vulnerability during labour [10, 11].

1.2.2 Doula support

The authors recognised professional doulas as specialised companions trained to provide continuous support during labour. Doulas assist with non-medical care, helping to reduce stress and offering comfort techniques, and are often linked with improved maternal outcomes [10, 12, 14].

1.2.3 Midwifery companionship

The authors noted midwifery companionship as a form that combines medical expertise with emotional support. This dual role helps mothers feel cared for holistically, contributing to positive birth experiences and enhancing the sense of safety [12, 14, 17].

1.2.4 Peer companionship

Peer companionship, including friends or community members, was identified by the authors as an informal but crucial form of support. Peers provide emotional closeness and familiarity, which can help reduce anxiety and create a sense of shared experience [11, 15].

1.2.5 Family member support

The authors discussed family member support, often from mothers or siblings, as another significant type of companionship. Family companions provide emotional bonding, cultural support, and practical assistance during labour, which can be particularly comforting for women [9, 11, 15]. The literature revealed issues to do with companionship having benefits to the pregnant outcome and emphasised physical presence, which is possible when the environment permits, but did not consider the low-resource income countries where there is no such space. Hence, the purpose of this study was to explore the meaning of companionship in a low-resource country.

1.3 Methodology

A study site is a natural setting where participants with characteristics describing the phenomenon under study are found [13, 16]; as such, this study was carried out between 15 and 30 September 2024 at a public health institution in a low-resource setup. The reason for choosing this setup is because it did not have space for allowing birth companions of choice to be with their loved ones in labour. The researchers wanted to understand what a birth companion meant to both the mothers and their carers and how the carers and labouring mothers practised the concept of companionship in labour, drawing from their experience in a setup where it is difficult to create a space for such to happen.

Purposive sampling is associated with detecting and engaging participants with features that enable them to address the study's aims [17–20]. A purposive sampling approach was used to obtain study participants with experience in the area of investigation [21]. A purposive sampling design was used, as it was ideal to choose participants with the required characteristics of the phenomenon of concern. The midwives working in the labour ward and those in the admission ward are the ones dealing with labouring mothers, and the mothers are the ones needing psychological and emotional support. Hence, both the mothers and the midwives' experiences would reveal what they experienced during their interactions in the context of companionship in labour in a difficult and unconducive set. The present study employed a phenomenological study to explore the experiences among postnatal women and their carers towards companionship in labour in a public hospital in a low-resource setup. Two focused group discussions were carried out: one with 10 healthcare workers, five from the labour ward and five from the admission ward. The second focus group discussion was carried out with eight postnatal mothers.

1.3.1 Recruitment of participants

The process of enrolment and fortifying informed consent comprised providing potential participants with a participant information sheet offering and debriefing on the aim of the study and informing participants why they have been selected [20], after which written consent was attained. The present study is qualitative, using a phenomenology design ideal for exploring experiences [19]. To select the participants into the study a selection criterion was set. That is for the midwives to qualify for the study they had to, working in maternity for two years, either working in the labour ward or admissions but were on duty when the women in the postnatal ward were labouring. The midwives who participated in the study were randomly selected using the duty roster as a sampling frame. The researchers wanted to understand and interpret the concept of 'Being and Time'. This appeared that this was ideal for the researchers to develop questions which were centered around having someone of choice during labour. For example, 'Tell me what it means to be with someone of choice being there for you whilst you were labouring' The flow of the conversion was determined by the responses which were coming up. This was to understand what these women think, feel and understand being accompanied in labour in a setting without the required resources and what it means to be in the situation at that particular point in time inherent in the individual's beliefs [19, 20].

1.4 Data collection

A phenomenological design permits specific ways of collecting data [19, 20, 22, 23]; a key method is semi-structured interviews, which the researcher implemented for the present study. In this instance, semi-structured interviews permitted further explanation of mothers' and their carer's experiences of implementing the companionship concept in an unconducive setting and the alternative strategies in such an environment, which could facilitate companionship in labour without compromising its benefit.

The reputation of interviews as a data collection instrument is founded on the strategies that produce accounts within a social setting, such as maternity wards, where this data was collected and perceived to represent the reality [22, 24] of companionship in a low-resource setting. As a result, the interviews generated real experiences of implementing companionship in labour from the participants' world [25]. The interviews are therefore assessed in association with the environment where data is generated about the possibility of implementing companionship in a low-resource setting, which is not conducive, and the culture revealed by participants' construct of reality [26, 27] and making the interviews appreciated as real instruments in data collection [28] in a social and natural setting of labour and delivery. Interviews are perceived as being influenced by social dynamics and cannot be divorced from the social context [29]; hence, they were a relevant data collection method for this study.

One topic guide was used to guide the Focused Group Discussions (FDGs) for both postnatal mothers and their carers to focus in-depth interviews on their experiences of implementing companionship in a low-resource setting [27, 30, 31]. The FDG for healthcare givers lasted 45 minutes, whilst that for postnatal women lasted 35 minutes. It is argued that the FDGs can be explored in the participants' beliefs, experiences, understandings, and inspirations concerning specific issues [32], such as that of companionship in labour in an unconducive setting. During the FDGs, the researchers penetrated superficial descriptions by probing changing topics, varying the omissions, and confirming earlier points that have been discussed. It appeared that the FDGs were helpful in that the collaborations among interviewees were very lively and produced very credible information. There was a lot of teamwork among the interviewees to such an extent that by the end of the 40-minute session, the same issues were coming up over and over again, which determined the stopping of the discussions. That transpired in all the two groups. According to Stewart and Shamdasani [33], guidelines received much attention to inspire all participants to dialogue and to contain individuals who tried to dominate the discussions. A clear benefit was that it assisted the researcher to mine data from various individuals in a short space of time. FGDs are a technique of generating qualitative data that involves a small group of people in a focused group conversation about a certain topic or collection of topics [34]. Companionship in labour this time. Hayward et al., Israel et al., and Cornwall and Jewkes [35–37] believe in FGDs as a technique whereby a researcher generates data from a group of individuals to debate on a specific topic, looking to gain an understanding of complex personal experiences, beliefs, perceptions, and attitudes related to a characteristic group of participants through a controlled interaction. Accordingly, FDGs are often utilised as a qualitative strategy to get an in-depth understanding of societal issues [38, 39]. The group frequently comprises of six to twelve people, depending on the researcher's assessment of the characteristics to be covered [40, 41]. Accordingly, for the two FDGs, the participants were selected from all the three shifts in order to explore whether the challenges were different for a specific shift.

1.4.1 Data collection process

To hold the weight on the issue at hand of companionship implementation challenges, the researcher created a focus group discussion topic guide that included a series of generic questions that sought responses to the researcher's queries. The researcher used a recorder for audiotaping and a form which presents issues for probing. The questions were all open-ended to permit the participants to freely elaborate their views as much as possible. Since most of the questions were designed by the researcher before getting into the field, there was a lot of refinement during the testing of the instrument as the reality of the FDGs evolved.

Before beginning the FGDs, the drive of the study and the process were elucidated to make the participant feel comfortable and relaxed, empowering them to deliberate their views without restrictions [21]. Such a tactic aided both the participants and the researcher to generate rapport and to enable the participants to offer their comprehensive understanding of companionship in labour and ensure the generation of quality data, as the researcher-participant relationship encompasses the real process of data collection [42]. The credibility of the questions lies in the questioning technique and the wording of the questions to be able to identify the participants' experiences and the motive behind their behaviour in addressing their challenges [34] related to employing the concept of companionship in labour. For example, the initial questions focused on the participant's knowledge of companionship in labour: "What do you know about companionship in labour? On views, "What are your views about on challenges faced in implementing companionship in labour for you?" and for practices. "Which skills do you think you have acquired for you to feel that you have benefited from companionship in labour?" and for social processes "Tell me about the social interactions which you were involved in to facilitate companioship during your time in labourward and / admission. The continuousness of the process relied on the individual's response [43–45]. The questions were expressed in such a way so as to be as neutral as possible [45]. However, the interview process worked through the mutual trust which had developed between the researcher and the participants. The researcher was conscious to the types of interrogations she enquired in an effort to motivate the participants to truly picture their thinking. Such a method is believed to yield worth and trustworthy information, which was the purpose of the present study [35] In the present study, the researcher wrote memos to capture any situation and idea rising during the research process [34]. According to [36]. Memos were written throughout the process and organised and to contain the date it was developed, an idea, hypothesis or question connected to their interview questions, emerged themes [21, 35] posits that, individuals react according to the meanings that they give to their acts and to the actions of others". This assisted the researcher in understanding various actions by different mothers and carers towards companionship in labour.

1.5 Data analysis

Guba [46] defines data analysis as an action of collating and unifying raw data in a way that facilitates the production of meaningful information. The main goal of carrying out a study is to translate data into findings. According to Merriam and Tisdell [47], qualitative research is inductive. Data analysis is a systematic process of ordering, bringing direction, and making sense out of the gathered data for informed decision-making [48, 49]. This study implemented a thematic data analysis approach, a qualitative data analysis method that includes reading through a data set and detecting upcoming themes [50]. Accordingly, Clarke and Braun [51] proposed a six-phase framework for undertaking a thematic analysis: Step 1: Becoming familiar with the data. Step 2 is to generate initial codes. Step 3: Search for themes. Step 4: Review themes. Step 5: Define themes. Step 6: Write-up. In relation to Bryman [20], areas of interest that resulted included socio-demographic factors, knowledge and awareness factors, attitudes and beliefs, perceptions, and service-related factors, and these need to be processed into workable themes in line with Clarke and Braun [51] as is presented below.

1.5.1 Step 1: Becoming familiar with data

To the first one, Bryman [20] adds that it requires the researcher to organise and prepare the data for analysis through transcribing interviews, optimally scanning material, and cataloguing each visual material, among others. In order to satisfy this step, the researcher scribbled notes from the postnatal mothers and the midwives' experiences in a notebook and also typed notes and transcribed verbatim of interviews done in the field. I also started to listen over and over again before transcribing, and this was done by three researchers and then, I read and reread the transcripts to familiarise myself and understand the issues coming up. At this stage, we also began to write down early impressions coming up from the data.

1.5.2 Step 2: Generation of initial codes

The second step, according to Clarke and Braun [51], is to generate initial codes. At this stage, the three researchers began to organise research data generated from the participants in a meaningful and systematic way. Volumes of data were reduced into very small chunks of meaning. The researchers used open *coding*, which allowed them to develop and modify codes as we worked through. This is opposed to pre-set codes, which are set before analysis and are fixed.

1.5.3 Step 3: Search for themes

Maguire and Delahunt [52] posit that a theme is a pattern that reveals characteristics of something significant or interesting about the data and/or research question. Braun and Clarke [53] elucidate that there are no hard and fast rules about what makes a theme. A theme is categorised by its significance. We examined the codes that arose, and some of them clearly fit together into a theme. For example, we had several codes that related to the 'definition of companionship', 'types of companionship', and 'benefits of companionship'. Alternative ways of companionships were collated into initial themes accordingly. By the end of this step, the codes had been organised into broader themes that seemed to say something specific about this research question. The themes were predominately descriptive as they described patterns in the data relevant to the research question.

1.5.4 Step 4: Review themes

In this stage, the researchers reviewed, modified, and developed the preliminary themes that were identified in the previous step. The aim was to understand whether these were meaningful and made sense, and the researcher also aimed to understand if the data was relevant. The researcher also worked on whether the themes were coherent and distinct from each other and also if there were themes within themes (subthemes).

1.5.5 Step 5: Define themes

This step entailed the final refinement of the themes and the aim, according to what Braun and Clarke [53] called to '. *identify the 'essence' of what each theme is about*.' In that regard, the researcher wanted to understand what each theme was saying and, if there were sub-themes, how they interacted and related to the main theme? And how do the themes relate to each other?

1.5.6 Step 6: The write-up

The researchers came up with various drafts collaboratively. The aim was to capture as much detail as possible from the research process. The 5 steps described above were very useful in getting to this stage. In addition to the production of this chapter, some journal articles will be generated from the research.

1.6 Findings

Four themes emerged from this study: 'The knowledge of companionship labour', which is described in terms of understanding what it is and the source of information; 'Alternatives ways of offering companionship in labour', 'Benefits of companionship', 'Evolving nature of the companionship in labor' of choice in labour, each with their own subthemes. All these themes showed their connectedness in that for one to talk about companionship in labour, they should be able to have the knowledge of the nature of the concept. This will make it possible to identify it through its characteristics. For the individual to choose or adapt to what is possible, one should be aware of the factors determining its applicability.

1.6.1 Knowledge towards companionship in labour

In this study, it has been revealed that both the pregnant women and midwives are aware that companionship in labour and birth is having someone chosen by the pregnant woman to give them support throughout labour. Knowing about what companionship in labour was about and the source where the information was received from. The mothers also indicated that the source and depth of knowledge is critical, and when some of these women receive information they perceive as inadequate, they look for it. If the information is of much interest to them, they can leave the place without seeking understanding and look for it somewhere to quench their curiosity. Besides, there are those mothers who rely more on the information the carers give them and get satisfied accordingly. Hence, it is revealed in this study that pregnant women get information from both the carers and the internet. As revealed in the following verbatim by PNW1 and PNW3, respectively.

> *'...Companionship in labour when a labouring woman is allowed ... having someone who assist to be able to go through labour without problems, I learnt about this from the antenatal clinic and read about it on internet,,,,, I got interested in it and I had not heard about it before, that's what I came to know more about it more.... in the antenatal clinic they do not give you much except that of having someone to be with you in labour.... And it part of quality care ...,' (PNW1)*

> *'What I know is that from the antenatal care clinic we were told that we can bring anyone we want to be with us when we get in labour but I don't know much about it ... and I am not sure whether I have said is correct.........." (PNW3)*

Knowing about companionship in labour among midwives is about understanding its purpose and learning about it. Being aware of the concept could be through capacity-building workshops and peer sharing. Some of the midwives defined it from a quality care perspective; besides having a companion of choice, they can also see it as part of respectful maternity care and a quality care measure, as revealed in the following two quotes, LMW2 and AdMW1, respectively.

> *Companionship is about the support the pregnant woman received from anyone whom they would have chosen to be with them throughout labour and to my understanding this is part of respectful maternity care I learnt about this from a capacity building workshop on Respectful Maternity Care workshop LMW2.*

> *What I know about companionship is about .... having someone by the side when in labour to encourage you pull through labour to make it tolerable and improve the quality of care .... According to what my colleagues taught me (AdMW1)*

1.6.2 The challenges associated with companionship in labour

The types of companionship emerged when the mothers and midwives were describing the challenges of space and provision of privacy and confidentiality, policy barring those accompanying those women in pregnancy; there were challenges of policy implementation associated with exclusion of companionship. The women, because of this policy, viewed it as violating their right to companionship. Violation of the companionship right emerged to be associated with pain and stress, as revealed in the following quote by *PNW2.*

> *When you come from home you are in pain and you are accompanied by your husband, mother sister or friend you are told they are not allowed in The moment you reach admissions you are asked to take your bags inside leaving the one who came with you outside. They are asked to go back home and come back during visiting us to check on where you have been admitted. Chasing my companion of choice is violating my rights, it stresses me making me anxious and angry. At least allow them to reach the admission door carrying my belongings and place them at the appropriate place. How painful and stressing to hear the security guard or the care giver chasing away someone who have accompanied you without even knowing your condition. (PNW2)*

Besides stress associated with policy, there is fear associated with being perceived as left alone. Though, at times the policy is flouted, the regulations are followed when the woman is accompanied by their mother.

As reflected in the following statement by PNW 3.

> *I came with my mother and she was allowed in labour ward and told not look at other patients as she got in carrying my belongings but I did not want her to leave me alone making me feel afraid of being alone (PNW3)*

With husbands being affected by the challenge of privacy as reflected in the following statements by PNW4 and AdMW 4, LMW, respectively.

> *Most of us we come with our husbands and find it is very difficult to let them in in the presence of other women who are naked '(PNW4)*

> *'Most of patients are naked......There is no room for that we do not have privacy the companions will violate the rights of other patients so we do not allow them they go*

> *home and come during visiting our just to check on where their patient is they will only see them after delivery…….'. (AdMW 4)*

> *'Most of patients are naked……. There is no room for that we do not have privacy in labour ward there are glasses which makes it possible for the client in the next cubicle peep will violate the rights of other people's wives so we do not practice companionship here ……. The husbands are asked to go home and come during visiting hour just to check on where their patient is they will only see them after delivery……. In post-natal'. (LMW5)*

Some challenges that emerged were associated with a shortage of staff, which needed the midwife to leave admissions unattended as they referred patients to the labour ward. The patients will then be expected to carry their bags, which at times is difficult because of pain. Due to this challenge, some midwives will allow the accompanying individuals to sit on the bench outside so that they can assist them with carrying patients' bags to labour and allow intermittent companionship as well.

> *'We were having problems with patients carrying their bags after sending those who accompanied the patients away and at times you are the only one here and you have to take the women to labour carrying their bags which they will put on the floor and respond to pain and pick it when the pain goes and takes longer to walk them to labour ward. We do not allow them in because the environment is not conducive …. They sit on the bench outside the admission entrance and then assist their relative to go to labour ward and sit at the foyer until their patient is made comfortable' (PNW 5)*

1.6.3 Alternative ways of implementing companionship in labour

The theme of alternative ways of implementing companionship in labour emerged when both the women and the midwives were discussing the challenges associated with offering companionship in labour.

1.6.3.1 Physical presence companionship in labour

When companionship is about having the individual with the mother throughout their labour, it is called physical presence. The issue of physical presence also appeared to be addressed through the phone and served the same purpose with an individual who is in close proximity, as reflected in the following statement by PNW 7.

> *Myself when I came to labour I was the only one in labour for a long time and when I got there my husband was allowed to stay with me …. We were put inside a curtain and was asked to wait outside when three other women came in an ambulance and that's when we got separated………..here I am alone …. but I was on the phone also showing him videos and he continued to reassure me and felt his presence (PNW7)*

However, it emerged in this study that if the environment permits physical presence in companionship, labour is possible and provides the necessary benefits. This is revealed in the following statement by PNW 5.

With my first baby I was in a private clinic ...... there was that privacy and we were left the two of us to feel our joy and pleasure of this journey together... I felt a genuine connection to my husband when I started labouring and he was with me rubbing my back listening to music together...., That feeling of being together combine with joy of shared experiences, contributes to the overall made me feel special the praise and shared information praise, information the. I was so relaxed that I did not notice that labour was over in n time. .... Felt calm and loved though its different now ...... here I am alone .... He brought me here and felt sad when he was leaving ......but promised to be with me (PNW 5)

1.6.4 Psychological presence companionship in labour

Psychological presence is about knowing that there is someone available who can be contacted if need be. The woman finds satisfaction in knowing that her labour companion has not been chased away. This happens when the labouring women accept that the environment does not allow their companion to be physically available for them. Even if they are to be chased away, at least this should happen with the woman not hearing it. That feeling alone will allay the anxiety and fear related to labour, producing the same effect with a companion who is present. This could be deemed as a complete psychological presence, as revealed in the following statement by PNW4.

At least do not chase them away whilst I hear give them some to sit so that at least in my mind I have the comfort of knowing that there is at least someone there for me nearby and they can be called if anything happens to me I have support nearby. We know that there is no private space for me to have my husband or partner in. That psychological presence is what is critical I will feel their presence even if they will go away but my brain will register that I have someone there for me (PNW4)

1.6.5 Intermittent presence companionship in labour

Intermittent presence companionship is associated with the combination of psychological and physical presence. This could be described on a continuum of physical-psychological presence. This means that at one point, the labour companion is there physically, and at one point, they are not with the labouring woman, but the labouring woman knows that they are nearby without even seeing them. The separation comes when the woman enters admissions for examination and comes together to share the results or is accompanied to the labour ward.

As reflected in the following statement by PNW 6.

At least allow them to be nearby so that when I come out of admissions I am able to talk to them and accompany me to labour ward carrying my things and give them to the labour ward midwife .... (PNW6)

Or if labour is not yet advanced, allow the woman to be with their companion outside admissions or the labour ward until a time she feels she needs to come back and be continuously monitored in labour. As revealed in the following statement

Allow me out of the examination room .... and allow me to go back to be with the person who have come with me if the labour is not to painful I will be coming in out and when the pain become severe I will come back PNW 1

> *Or the companion sits in the labour ward foyer where the woman will be moving in and out of the labour ward to be with their companion, as reflected in the following statement by AdMW2*

> *' It depends on who is there for me I allow the companion to sit on the bench and allow the woman to move in and out as long as they are able to do so until they are seen and then then to labour ward I can either carry the bags or ask the relatives to carry the bag to labour ward... and can wait as long as they can in the labour ward foyer* **(AdMW2)**

1.6.6 Transit companionship in labour

The study results also revealed the accompaniment associated with being with the woman as they are on their way to the labour ward and block the one accompanying the woman at the door. This type of companionship in labour only occurs outside the institution. Blocking the person accompanying the women in labour is described by women as a violation of their rights to quality care and likened to chasing away companions and the most stressful scenario, as revealed in the following statement by PNW 2.

> *When you come from home you are in pain and you are accompanied by your husband, mother sister or friend, the moment you reach admissions you are asked to take your bags inside leaving the one who came with you outside. They are asked to go back home and come back during visiting us to check on where you have been admitted. Chasing my companion of choice is violating my rights. At least allow them to reach the admission door carrying my belongings and place them at the appropriate place. How painful and stressing to hear the security guard or the care giver chasing away someone who have accompanied you without even knowing your condition. (PNW2)*

1.6.7 Benefits of companionship

According to this study, there are several benefits of companionship in labour, such as promoting patient relaxation, feeling empowered, alleviating anxiety, and building trust in the environment. As reflected in the following statement by PNW5.

> *With my first baby I was in a private clinic ...... there was that privacy and we were left the two of us to feel our joy and pleasure of this journey together.... I felt a genuine connection to my husband when I started labouring and he was with me rubbing my back listening to music together...., That feeling of being together combine with joy of shared experiences, contributes to the overall made me feel special the praise and shared information praise, information the. I was so relaxed that I did not notice that labour was over in n time. .... Felt calm and loved though its different now ...... here I am alone .... He brought me here and felt sad when he was leaving ......but promised to be with me, he would talk to nurses and doctor on my behalf and facilitated my understanding where I missed or not understand explanations (PNW 5)*

In this study, it emerged that companionship is associated with a feeling of safety, relaxation and protection, as revealed in the following statement by PNW 1 and LMW4, respectively.

I Felt safe, relaxed and protected when I had my mother with me in labour (PNW 1)

I have observed that when labour ward is not busy and allow the women to be with their companions the woman is very happy and even talking and laughing together but the moment the companion goes they start crying and seeking attention from you... when you get in the cubicle they are quiet and what you to hold their hand rub their back and stay with them. (LMW4)

1.7 Discussion

1.7.1 Psychosocial characteristics of companionship in labour

Companionship has been viewed as the most powerful component of respectful maternity care, which improves the quality of labour and birth management in pregnant women. Similarly, both the postnatal women and midwives acknowledge that accompaniment reduces stress and provides emotional support [4, 11, 12, 14, 15], communication support [4, 11, 12, 14–16], decision-making [4], and pain management [12, 14, 16], which emerged as psychological support, which includes increased satisfaction with labour [12, 14, 16]. Hence, it could be concluded that the concept of a labour companion has to do with psychosocial concepts as revealed in the literature and the present study.

1.7.2 Benefit of labour companion

The benefits that emerged in this study appear to be matched to those already known in the literature, which are matched with its psychosocial characteristics [9–12, 14, 15].

1.7.3 The impact of environment on implementation of companions in labour

In this study, it has emerged there were challenges with implementing companionship due to the type of environment the woman is labouring in. It appeared that the environment poses challenges, which forces those involved to come up with mitigatory strategies. These new approaches to implementing companionship in labour brought up the issues with presence being critical, issues to do with physical presence, which involved a complete accompaniment where the person accompanying the pregnant woman is defined by being there throughout labour and delivery. The issue of physical presence has been described in literature [5–12].

The present study brought up the concept of 'psychological presence' for the first time in literature. Though the concept of psychological presence emerged to bring similar effects when the labouring woman is able to continuously communicate with their companion on the phone and have video calls. Whilst the issue of the woman not being able to be with the labouring woman. Similarly, when the woman is psychologically and emotionally attached to their labour companion, the benefit is similar to that of physical presence, and this could be facilitated through voice and video calls. In this study, there emerged the framework of psychological presences which describes the interrelatedness of companionship implementation from a physical and psychological perspective on a continuum of physical and psychological presence companionship (intermittent companionship, transit companionship).

1.8 Contribution of this study

- Companion in labour is about sharing emotions and feelings between the pregnant woman and someone concerned about them.
- The study created a labour companion framework.
- Voice and voice call with a companion of choice is an effective labour companion.

Limitations of the study

The study used a single research site to represent the low-income setting and needs to be carried out on a larger scale.

Declaration of interest

The researchers have no interests to declare.

This study was sponsored by the block allocation fund from the Women's University in Africa research board fund.

Author details

Unice Goshomi*, Owen Goshomi and Angelline Goshomi
Women University in Africa, Harare, Zimbabwe

*Address all correspondence to: ugoshomi@yahoo.com

References

[1] Jacob A. A Comprehensive Textbook of Midwifery & Gynecological Nursing. New Dehli: Jaypee Brothers Medical Publishers; 2018

[2] Marshall JE. Myles Professional Studies for Midwifery Education and Practice: Concepts and Challenges. UK: Elsevier Health Sciences; 2019

[3] Mon NO. Labour companionship and women's experiences of mistreatment during childbirth: Results from a multi-country community-based survey. BMJ Global Health. 2022;5(Suppl 2):e003564

[4] Afulani PA, Okiring J, Aborigo RA, Nutor JJ, Kuwolamo I, Dorzie JBK, et al. Provider implicit and explicit bias in person-centered maternity care: A cross-sectional study with maternity providers in northern Ghana. BMC Health Services Research. 2023;**23**(1):254

[5] Lüscher BP, Schoeberlein A, Surbek DV, Baumann MU. Hyperuricemia during pregnancy leads to a preeclampsia-like phenotype in mice. Cells. 2022;**11**(22):3703

[6] Batra K, Singh TP, Sharma M, Batra R, Schvaneveldt N. Investigating the psychological impact of COVID-19 among healthcare workers: A meta-analysis. International Journal of Environmental Research and Public Health. 2020;**17**(23):9096

[7] AlKhunaizi AN, Al-Otaibi AG, Alharbi MF, Bahari G. Exploring healthcare providers' and Women's perspectives of labor companionship during childbirth: An interpretative phenomenological analysis study. In: Healthcare. Vol. 12. MDPI; 2024. p. 869

[8] Holopainen A, Hakulinen T. New parents' experiences of postpartum depression: A systematic review of qualitative evidence. JBI Evidence Synthesis. 2019;**17**(9):1731-1769

[9] Yaya Bocoum F, Kabore CP, Barro S, Zerbo R, Tiendrebeogo S, Hanson C, et al. Women's and health providers' perceptions of companionship during labor and childbirth: A formative study for the implementation of WHO companionship model in Burkina Faso. Reproductive Health. 2023;**20**(1):46

[10] Waterhouse B, O'Connor RJ. Care by companionship–a proposal for prescription friends. Journal of the Royal Society of Medicine. 2009;**102**(12):504-504

[11] Ashish KC. Co-designing interventions for a continuum of care for children with cerebral palsy. Developmental Medicine and Child Neurology. Aug 2024;**66**(8):971-972. DOI: 10.1111/dmcn.15848. Epub 2024 Jan 18

[12] Summerton JV, Mtileni TR, Moshabela ME. Experiences and perceptions of birth companions supporting women in labour at a district Hospital in Limpopo, South Africa. Curationis. 2021;**44**(1):2186

[13] Kiti G, Prata N, Afulani PA. Continuous labor support and person-centered maternity care: A cross-sectional study with women in rural Kenya. Maternal and Child Health Journal. 2022;**26**(1):205-216

[14] Summerton JV, Mtileni T. Birth companion of choice: A survey amongst women who have given birth at a rural hospital in Limpopo, South Africa. International Journal of Pregnancy & Child Birth. 2020;**6**(6):148-153

[15] Ashish KC. Hospital care among children with chronic illness during the COVID-19 pandemic in England. Evidence-Based Nursing. 2023;**26**(3):98-98

[16] Jayasundara DMCS, Jayawardane IA, Weliange SDS, Jayasingha TDKM, Madugalle TMSSB. Impact of continuous labor companion-who is the best: A systematic review and meta-analysis of randomized controlled trials. PLoS One. 2024;**19**(7):e0298852

[17] Beyene K, Fekadu K, Yihune M, Alemayehu Y, Alelign D, Ashebir G, et al. Decision to delivery interval, perinatal outcome and factors following emergency cesarean section in southern Ethiopia. Ethiopian Journal of Health Sciences. 2023;**33**(1):39-48

[18] Polit DF, Beck CT. Essentials of Nursing Research: Appraising Evidence for Nursing Practice. NY: Lippincott Williams & Wilkins; 2010

[19] Strauss A, Corbin J. Basics of Qualitative Research Techniques. Thousand Oaks, CA: Sage Publications; 1998

[20] Cresswell J. Qualitative Inquiry & Research Design: Choosing among Five Approaches. Thousand Oaks, CA. Sage Publications; 2013

[21] Creswell JW, Plano-Clark VL. Designing and Conducting Mixed Methods Research. Thousand Oaks, Calif: SAGE Publications; 2007

[22] Bryman A. Social Research Methods. Oxford, UK: Oxford University Press; 2016

[23] Gallagher S. What is phenomenology? In: Phenomenology. Cham: Springer International Publishing; 2022. pp. 1-10

[24] Goldblatt H, Karnieli-Miller O, Neumann M. Sharing qualitative research findings with participants: Study experiences of methodological and ethical dilemmas. Patient Education and Counseling. 2011;**82**(3):389-395

[25] Hammersley M. Interview data: A qualified defence against the radical critique. Qualitative Research. 2017;**17**(2):173-186

[26] Murphy L, Lewandowski G, McCauley R, Simon B, Thomas L, Zander C. Debugging: The good, the bad, and the quirky--A qualitative analysis of novices' strategies. ACM SIGCSE Bulletin. 2008;**40**(1):163-167

[27] Mason J. Researching your Own Practice: The Discipline of Noticing. London, UK: Routledge; 2002

[28] Maxwell JA. Qualitative Research Design: An Interactive Approach: An Interactive Approach. Carlifornia, USA: Sage; 2013

[29] Fontana A, Frey JH. The interview. The Sage Handbook of Qualitative Research. 2005;**3**(1):695-727

[30] Brinkmann S, Kvale S. Confronting the ethics of qualitative research. Journal of Constructivist Psychology. 2005;**18**(2):157-181

[31] Green J, Thorogood N. Analysing qualitative data. In: Principles of Social Research. Open University Press; 2005. pp. 75-89

[32] Gill TK, Tucker GR, Avery JC, Shanahan EM, Menz HB, Taylor AW, et al. The use of self-report questions to examine the prevalence of musculoskeletal problems: A test-retest study. BMC Musculoskeletal Disorders. 2016;**17**:1-10

[33] Stewart DW, Shamdasani PN. Focus Groups: Theory and Practice. Vol. 20. Carlifornia, USA: Sage Publications; 2014

[34] Wilkinson S. Focus groups. In: Doing Social Psychology Research. Oxford: Blackwell Publishing Ltd.; 2004. pp. 344-376

[35] Hayward M, Awenat Y, McCarthy Jones S, Paulik G, Berry K. Beyond beliefs: A qualitative study of people's opinions about their changing relations with their voices. Psychosis. 2015;*7*(2):97-107

[36] Israel BA, Schulz AJ, Parker EA, Becker AB. Review of community-based research: Assessing partnership approaches to improve public health. Annual Review of Public Health. 1998;**19**(1):173-202

[37] Cornwall A, Jewkes R. What is participatory research? Social Science & Medicine. 1995;**41**(12):1667-1676

[38] Nyumba T O, Wilson K, Derrick CJ, Mukherjee N. The use of focus group discussion methodology: Insights from two decades of application in conservation. Methods in Ecology and Evolution. 2018;**9**(1):20-32

[39] Dockett S, Perry B, Kearney E. Promoting children's informed assent in research participation. International Journal of Qualitative Studies in Education. 2013;**26**(7):802-828

[40] Morgan DL. Basic and Advanced Focus Groups. CA, USA: Sage Publications; 2018

[41] Morgan DL. Qualitative content analysis: A guide to paths not taken. Qualitative Health Research. 1993;**3**(1):112-121

[42] Aguas PP. Fusing approaches in educational research: Data collection and data analysis in phenomenological research. The Qualitative Report. 2022;**27**(1):1-20

[43] Charmaz K. Grounded theory in global perspective: Reviews by international researchers. Qualitative Inquiry. 2014;**20**(9):1074-1084

[44] Glaser B, Bailyn L, Fernandez W, Holton JA, Levina N. What grounded theory is.... In: Academy of Management Proceedings. Vol. 1. Briarcliff Manor, NY: Academy of Management; 2013. p. 11290

[45] Artinian BM, Giske T, Cone PH, editors. Glaserian Grounded Theory in Nursing Research: Trusting Emergence. NY: Springer Publishing Company; 2009

[46] Guba EG. Competing paradigms in qualitative research. In: Handbook of Qualitative Research. Sage; 1994

[47] Merriam SB, Tisdell EJ. Qualitative Research: A Guide to Design and Implementation. USA: John Wiley & Sons; 2015

[48] Silverman D. Interpreting qualitative data. Organization Studies-Berlin-European Group For Organizational Studies. 2002;**23**(1):161-161

[49] Miles MB, Huberman AM, Saldaña J. Qualitative Data Analysis: A Methods Sourcebook. 3rd ed. CA, USA: Sage Publications; 2014

[50] Rahman MS. The advantages and disadvantages of using qualitative and quantitative approaches and methods in language "testing and assessment" research: A literature review. Journal of Education and Learning. 2016;**6**(1):102-112

[51] Clarke V, Braun V. Thematic analysis. The Journal of Positive Psychology. 2017;**12**(3):297-298

[52] Maguire M, Delahunt B. Doing a thematic analysis: A practical, step-by-step guide for learning and teaching scholars. All Ireland Journal of Higher Education. 2017;**9**(3):33501-33513

[53] Braun V, Clarke V. Using thematic analysis in psychology. Qualitative Research in Psychology. 2006;**3**(2):77-101

Chapter 4

Disrespect and Abuse during Childbirth in Public Health Facilities, Ethiopia

Ahmedin Aliyi Usso

Abstract

Maternal mortality and morbidity can be significantly reduced by providing compassionate and respectful care during childbirth. However, there is limited information on the prevalence of disrespect and abuse during childbirth in eastern Ethiopia. This study aimed to assess the level of disrespect and abuse experienced by women who gave birth in public health facilities in eastern Ethiopia. The study found that 77% of women who gave birth at public health facilities in eastern Ethiopia experienced disrespect and abuse during childbirth. Encouraging all pregnant women to attend antenatal care visits and enhancing the quality of health care services provided at night in all health facilities would be critical for preventing and mitigating disrespect and abuse, as well as their negative implications.

Keywords: disrespect and abuse, respectful maternity care, childbirth, health facilities, Ethiopia

1. Introduction

Respectful maternity care, which includes dignity, privacy, and confidentiality, is a fundamental human right for every woman across all healthcare facilities. This type of care ensures informed choices and continuity of healthcare while safeguarding women from harm and mistreatment [1, 2]. It is a crucial aspect of quality maternity care [3]. Disrespectful and abusive treatment toward women during childbirth is a violation of their human rights. It can negatively impact institutional birth coverage [1, 4], leading to increased risks of maternal and newborn mortality, particularly in sub-Saharan African countries (SSA).

While the proportion of births attended by skilled professionals has improved in higher-income countries over the past decade, low- and middle-income countries (LMICs) still have low coverage of skilled birth attendance [5, 6]. For instance, in 2018, the global proportion of skilled birth attendance was 81%, with almost 100% in higher-income countries, 82% in Southeast Asia, 60% in sub-Saharan Africa (SSA), and only 48% in Ethiopia [6, 7]. Poor quality services and mistreatment by healthcare providers in facilities may contribute to the low coverage of skilled birth attendance [8, 9].

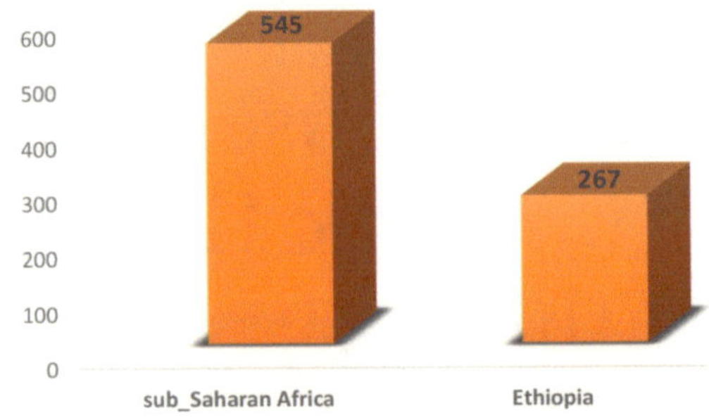

Figure 1.
Maternal mortality ratio per 100,000 live births in sub-Saharan Africa and Ethiopia.

Maternal mortality is a significant public health issue in developing countries, especially in sub-Saharan Africa (SSA) [10]. Ensuring the presence of skilled birth attendants during childbirth is a crucial strategy for preventing and reducing maternal mortality in these countries [11–13]. According to data from 2020, approximately 287,000 maternal deaths occurred annually in the world due to birth-related complications, with 95% of these deaths occurring in low- and middle-income countries (LMICs). More than 70% of these deaths, amounting to 545 per 100,000 live births, occurred in SSA, and 267 maternal deaths per 100,000 live births were recorded in Ethiopia in 2020 [14] shown in **Figure 1**. The higher rates of maternal mortality in these regions were associated with low rates of skilled birth attendance in developing countries [6, 10].

The Ethiopian government's health sector transformation plan based on the sustainable development goals (SDGs) aims to reduce maternal mortality to 70 per 100,000 by 2030 [15, 16]. Achieving this target requires improving the quality of maternal healthcare services by providing respectful maternity care at every woman's interaction with health facilities [17]. Improving respectful maternity care has been identified as a potential strategy to prevent and reduce maternal mortality, which can be accomplished by increasing the coverage of skilled birth attendance [3, 18].

2. Disrespect and abuse during childbirth

Respectful and abusive behavior during childbirth are serious violations of women's human rights and a sign of substandard care. Factors contributing to this issue include challenging circumstances in the healthcare system and the sociocultural environment that enables such behavior. Providers may resort to disrespectful and abusive tactics when feeling overwhelmed and powerless, as reported by one study [19].

Disrespect and abusive behavior during childbirth in healthcare facilities may include physical abuse, extreme humiliation, and verbal abuse, as well as unapproved medical procedures, lack of confidentiality, inadequate informed consent, denial of pain relief, serious breaches of privacy, refusal of admission to healthcare facilities, neglect leading to life-threatening complications, and detention of women and their newborns due to inability to pay [20].

2.1 Adverse effects of disrespect and abuse during childbirth

Disrespect and abuse can have several detrimental effects.

- It can be a violation of human rights that undermines women's citizenship and autonomy.
- It can reduce satisfaction and trust in the healthcare system, ultimately resulting in unfavorable health outcomes.
- It can have a direct impact on adverse health outcomes.
- It can have negative economic consequences [21].

2.2 Respectful maternity care

It is important to realize that the absence of disrespect and abuse during childbirth does not equal respectful maternity care; instead, high-quality, woman-centered care requires intentional effort and should be a top priority for healthcare providers and systems [22, 23]. To this end, advocates have called for respectful care and protection for all childbearing women, especially those who are marginalized and vulnerable, such as adolescents, ethnic and racial minorities, and women with disabilities. The Respectful Maternity Care movement typically promotes a patient-centered approach grounded in respect for women's basic human rights and supported by clinical evidence.

There are seven rights that women have during childbearing:

- Freedom from harm and mistreatment
- Access to information, informed consent, and the ability to make choices, including the right to choose a support person whenever possible
- Confidentiality and privacy
- Dignity and respect
- Equality, freedom from discrimination, and equitable care
- Timely healthcare and the highest attainable level of health
- Liberty, autonomy, self-determination, and freedom from coercion (See **Table 1**) [23].

2.3 Impact of disrespect and abuse during childbirth

The extent of disrespect and abuse in eastern Ethiopia was 77.0%, with similar levels observed in Addis Ababa (78%), and 98.9% in Arba Minch, Southern Ethiopia, Wollega, Eastern Ethiopia, and western Ethiopia (74.8%) [24, 25]. In the Oromia

Reported types of disrespect and abuse during childbirth	Frequency (n)	Percentage (%)
1. Physical abuse	**142**	**26.8**
Health provider physically hit or slapped mother	99	18.7
Health provider verbally insulted mother	120	22.6
Care provider separate mother from baby without indication	50	9.4
Supportive staff insult mother and her companion	50	9.4
Provider denied mother from food or fluid without indication	89	16.8
Providers did not permit mother to choose a position for birth	96	19.1
2. Non-confidential care	**252**	**47.5**
Care providers did not use covering to protect mother privacy	177	33.4
Providers discussed mother's privacy in a way other could hear	105	19.8
3. Non-informed consent care	**259**	**48.9**
Provider did not introduce himself/herself to mother	259	48.9
Providers did not explain the findings of mothers'	67	12.6
Providers did not explain to mother what is done and to expect	67	12.6
Providers did not encourage the mother to ask questions	86	16.2
Provider did not respond to mother's question with politeness	99	18.7
Provider did not obtain consent before a procedure	233	44.0
4. Non-dignified care	**135**	**25.5**
Health providers shout at or intimidate mother	135	25.5
Health providers made negative comment about mother	111	20.9
Providers not allowed mother's companion into delivery room	115	21.5
5. Abandonment of care	**53**	**10.0**
Providers ignored or abandoned mother when called for help	53	10
Mother gave birth alone because providers not present	11	2.1
6. Discrimination	**29**	**5.5**
Provider discriminates against mother by educational or economic status	29	5.5
Provider discriminates against mother by resident area	16	3.0
Providers discriminate against mother because of her age	10	1.9
7. Detention in health facilities	**13**	**2.5**
Mother's discharge postponed until facility bills paid	9	1.7
Mother detained in a health facility due to the damage to the property	4	0.8

Table 1.
Seven categories of disrespect and abuse with respective verification criteria.

region Bale zone, the prevalence of disrespect and abuse was 37.5%, 17.5% in Addis Ababa, and 67.1% in Bahir Dar, Amhara regional state (**Figure 2**) [26–30].

Among women who experienced disrespect and abuse, non-informed consent care (48.9%) was the most common category, with the provider not introducing themselves to the woman and her companion (48.9%) being the most frequently reported form of disrespect and abuse. The second most common category was non-confidential care (47.5%), with 33.4% of women reporting that care providers did not use a drape or cover to protect their privacy. Physical abuse (26.8%) was the third most common category, followed by non-dignified care (25.5%), abandonment care (10.0%), discrimination (5.5%), and detention (2.5%), as summarized in **Table 1**.

Factors such as women's sociocultural status, attitude toward maternity care, and health facilities' infrastructural problems may contribute to the increased prevalence of disrespect and abuse. For example, the number of institutional deliveries has increased in rural eastern Ethiopia without corresponding increases in infrastructure, staff, and supplies that could compromise respectful maternity care.

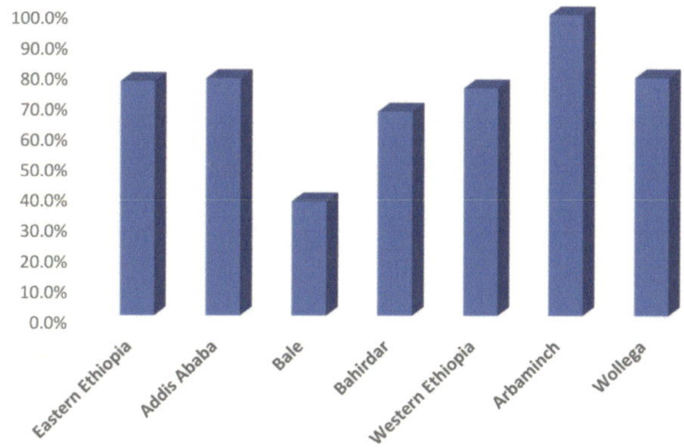

Figure 2.
Prevalence of disrespect and abuse during childbirth in Ethiopian regions.

2.4 Factors associated with disrespect and abuse during childbirth

The economic status of women often acts as a significant deterrent to receiving compassionate and respectful maternity care in public health facilities. Research has shown that women with lower incomes are more likely to experience disrespect and abuse during childbirth, even more so than women with higher incomes [24, 25, 28, 31, 32]. This is likely because providers tend to prioritize women with higher incomes over those with lower incomes, leading to care being provided to affluent women before poor women, regardless of the severity of their medical condition [25, 33].

Women who live far from public health facilities are also more likely to experience disrespect and abuse during childbirth. This could be due to these women having limited knowledge, involvement, and decision-making abilities, making them passive and powerless in the care they receive. It is crucial to address this issue and ensure that all women, regardless of their location, receive respectful maternity care during childbirth. Improving the quality and access to healthcare services is an important step toward achieving this goal [34].

Furthermore, women with a lower parity level of less than or equal to four are 1.7 times more likely to experience disrespect and abuse during childbirth in health facilities [34, 35]. Multiparous women, on the other hand, are more familiar with maternity care services provided in health facilities and may request missed services during childbirth.

According to the studies, women in Ethiopia who missed ANC visits during their pregnancies were more likely to be mistreated and abused during childbirth [26, 34, 36]. Proper use of maternity care services can raise women's knowledge of the healthcare system and provide them with the ability to protect themselves from mistreatment and violence during labor. Furthermore, punctuality for ANC visits may foster a close relationship between caregivers and patients. To prevent abuse during childbirth in healthcare facilities, all pregnant women must have access to ANC visits.

Women who gave birth at night were more likely to be disrespected and abused than those who gave birth during the day [34, 35, 37, 38]. It suggests that women who gave birth during the day were more likely to receive respectful maternity care than those who gave birth at night. This could be a shortage of care providers assigned during the night, leading to healthcare providers becoming overworked [38]. Additionally, there might be a tendency to provide poor-quality maternity care

Variables	Categories	Disrespected and abused		Adjusted OR (95% CI)
		Yes, n (%)	No, n (%)	
Residence area	Urban	77 (60.2)	51 (39.8)	1
	Rural	331 (82.3)	71 (17.7)	1.33 (0.65, 2.72)
Age (in year)	18–24	146 (83.0)	30 (17.0)	1.78 (0.71, 4.42)
	25–34	226 (76.1)	71 (23.9)	1.58 (0.74, 3.34)
	≥35	36 (63.2)	21 (36.8)	1
Monthly income (in USD)	<57.22	238 (87.5)	34 (12.5)	2.29 (1.41, 3.71) ***
	≥57.22	170 (65.9)	88 (34.1)	1
Distance from nearby health facility	≤30 minutes	94 (60.3)	62(39.7)	1
	>30 minutes	314 (84.0)	60(16.0)	2.10 (1.30, 3.39) **
Types of health facility	Health center	339 (78.1)	95 (21.9)	1.07 (0.60, 1.92)
	Hospital	69 (71.9)	27 (28.1)	1
Parity	≤4	313 (78.4)	86 (21.6)	1.70 (1.02, 2.84) *
	>4	95 (72.5)	36 (27.5)	1
Spontaneous vaginal delivery	Yes	338 (76.6)	103 (23.4)	0.88 (0.46, 1.70)
	No	70 (78.7)	19 (21.3)	1
Fetal birth outcome	Alive	380 (76.5)	117 (23.5)	1
	Dead	28 (84.8)	5 (15.2)	1.01 (0.32, 3.15)
Antenatal care attendance	Yes	262 (70.2)	111 (29.8)	1
	No	146 (93.0)	11 (7.0)	4.29 (2.17, 8.52) ***
Delivery time	Daytime	101 (62.7)	60 (37.3)	1
	Nighttime	307 (83.2)	62 (16.8)	2.16 (1.37, 3.41) ***
Gender of main birth attendance	Male	203 (77.2)	60 (22.8)	1.15 (0.73, 1.81)
	Female	205 (76.8)	62 (23.2)	1

*$p < 0.05$.
**$p < 0.01$.
***$p < 0.001$.

Table 2.
Factors associated with disrespect and abuse during childbirth. Multivariable analysis.

during the night due to the low number of staff members available for obstetric cases during the night shift [39]. Other challenges during the night include infrastructural problems, such as electricity interruptions [40, 41], which can impact the ability to receive respectful maternity care. It is concerning that women who attend the labor ward at night are more likely to be disrespected and abused. It is important to ensure respectful maternity care during the night by increasing the number of care providers assigned and implementing supervision during the night in all health facilities (**Table 2**).

3. Disrespect and abuse measurement

A study was conducted at several public health facilities in eastern Ethiopia. The study included 530 women who had given birth at these facilities. Disrespect and abuse are measured according to Bowser and Hill's framework and categorized into seven domains, including physical abuse, non-confidential care, non-informed consent, non-dignified care, abandonment of care, discrimination, and detention.

Each domain had multiple verification criteria, with dichotomous (yes/no) responses to measure the seven categories. Then, the woman is considered to have experienced disrespect and abuse if she responded 'Yes' to at least one of the seven verification criteria [20, 24, 25]. The prevalence of each of the seven categories of disrespect and abuse, with 24 items, is summarized in **Table 1**.

4. Conclusion

More than three in every four women who give birth in public health facilities in Ethiopia reported experiencing some form of disrespect and abuse throughout the process. Factors such as average monthly income, distance from nearby health facilities, attending ANC visits, and giving birth at night were significantly associated with disrespect and abuse. Encouraging all pregnant women to attend ANC checkups and increasing the quality of healthcare treatment at night in all health facilities by assigning appropriate staff and refilling supplies is critical for decreasing and preventing disrespect and abuse. In addition, specific strategies and interventions should be designed to ensure equitable access to quality maternity care during childbirth for women living far from health facilities.

Acknowledgements

I am pleased with the invitation to contribute to this chapter from Intech Open, an open-access publisher of books and journals. Additionally, I would like to express my gratitude to the publication process manager, Kristina Kardum Cvitan, for her constant assistance and direction during the writing process of this chapter.

Conflict of interest

The author declares no conflict of interest.

Author details

Ahmedin Aliyi Usso
College of Health and Medical Sciences, Haramaya University, Harar, Ethiopia

*Address all correspondence to: ahmedinfoan@gmail.com

References

[1] World Health Organization. The Prevention and Elimination of Disrespect and Abuse during Facility-Based Childbirth. Geneva: WHO, HNN Team; 2017

[2] World Health Organization. WHO Recommendations Intrapartum Care for a Positive Childbirth Experience. Geneva: World Health Organization; 2018

[3] Sheferaw ED, Mengesha TZ, Wase SB. Development of a tool to measure women's perception of respectful maternity care in public health facilities. BMC Pregnancy and Childbirth. 2016;**16**:67

[4] World Health Organization. Quality of Care for Maternal and Newborn Health: A Monitoring Framework for Network Countries. Genève, Switzerland: WHO; 2019

[5] Bohren MA, Vogel JP, Hunter EC, Lutsiv O, Makh SK, Souza JP. The mistreatment of women during childbirth in health facilities globally: A mixed-methods systematic review. PLOS Medicine. 2015;**12**(6):e1001847

[6] World Health Statistics. Monitoring Health for the SDGs, Sustainable Development Goals. Geneva: World Health Organization; 2019

[7] Ethiopia Mini Demographic and Health Survey (EMDHS). Ethiopian Public Health Institute (EPHI) [Ethiopia] and ICF. Ethiopia Mini Demographic and Health Survey 2019: Key Indicators. Vol. 2019. Rockville, Maryland, USA: EPHI and ICF; 2019

[8] Iloh G, Ofoedu J, Njoku P, Odu F, Ifedigbo C, Iwuamanam K. Evaluation of patients' satisfaction with quality of care provided at the National Health Insurance Scheme clinic of a tertiary hospital in South-Eastern Nigeria. Nigerian Journal of Clinical Practice. 2012;**15**(4):469-474

[9] Okafor I, Ugwu EO, Obi SN. Disrespect and abuse during facility-based childbirth in a low-income country. International Journal of Gynecology & Obstetrics. 2015;**128**(2):110-113

[10] WHO, UNICEF U, WB. Trends in maternal mortality: 1990 to 2015. In: WHO U, UNFPA, World Bank Group and the United Nations Population Division, editor. Trends in Maternal Mortality: 1990 to 2015. Geneva: WHO; 2015

[11] Amouzou A, Ziqi M, Carvajal-Aguirre L, Quinley J. Skilled attendant at birth and newborn survival in sub–Saharan Africa. Journal of Global Health. 2017;**7**(2):020504

[12] Goldenberg RL, McClure EM, Saleem S. Improving pregnancy outcomes in low-and middle-income countries. Reproductive Health. 2018;**15**(1):7-14

[13] Nyfløt L, Sitras V. Strategies to reduce global maternal mortality. Acta Obstetricia et Gynecologica Scandinavica. 2018;**97**(6):639-640

[14] World Health Organization. Trends in Estimates of Maternal Mortality Ratio (MMR; Maternal Deaths per 100,000 Live Births) Maternal Deaths and Lifetime Risk of Maternal Death, 2000-2020. In: WHO U, UNFPA, World Bank Group and UNPD (MMEIG) editor.: Geneva, Switzerland: World Health Organization; 2023.

[15] The Federal Democratic Republic of Ethiopia Ministry of Health (FMOH).

Health Sector Transformation Plan (2015/16-2019/20). Addis Ababa, Ethiopia: FMOH; 2015

[16] World Health Organization. SDG target 3.1, maternal mortality by 2030, reduce the global maternal mortality ratio to less than 70 per 100 000 live births. In: World Health Statistics 2023. Genève, Switzerland: World Health Organization; 2023

[17] Chukwuma A, Wosu AC, Mbachu C, Weze K. Quality of antenatal care predicts retention in skilled birth attendance: A multilevel analysis of 28 African countries. BMC Pregnancy and Childbirth. 2017;**17**:152

[18] World Health Organization. Strategies towards Ending Preventable Maternal Mortality (EPMM). Genève, Switzerland: World Health Organization; 2015

[19] World Health Organization. The Prevention and Elimination of Disrespect and Abuse during Facility-Based Childbirth. Geneva: World Health Organization; 2014

[20] Bowser D, Hill K. Exploring Evidence for Disrespect and Abuse in Facility-Based Childbirth: Report of a Landscape Analysis. Genève, Switzerland: USAID/TRAction Project; 2010

[21] World Health Organization. The Prevention and Elimination of Disrespect and Abuse during Facility-Based Childbirth. Geneva: WHO; 2015

[22] Amnesty International. Deadly Delivery: The Maternal Health Care Crisis in the USA. London: Amnesty International Secretariat; 2010

[23] White Ribbon Alliance. Respectful Maternity Care Charter. Genève, Switzerland: White Ribbon Alliance; 2011

[24] Asefa A, Bekele D. Status of respectful and non-abusive care during facility-based childbirth in a hospital and health centers in Addis Ababa, Ethiopia. Reproductive Health. 2015;**12**:33

[25] Tekle BF, Kebebe KH, Etana B, Woldie M, Feyissa TR. Disrespect and abuse during childbirth in Western Ethiopia: Should women continue to tolerate? PLoS One. 2019;**14**(6):e0217126

[26] Mekonnen A, Fikadu G, Esmeal A. Disrespectful and abusive maternity care during childbirth in bale zone public hospitals, Southeast Ethiopia: Cross sectional study. Clinical Practice. 2019;**16**(5):1273-1280

[27] Kitaw M, Tessema M. Respectful maternity care and associated factors among mothers in the immediate post-partum period, in public health facilities of Addis Ababa. International Journal of Pregnancy Child Birth. 2019;**5**(1):10-17

[28] Wassihun B, Deribe L, Worede N, Gultie T. Prevalence of disrespect and abuse of women during child birth and associated factors in Bahir Dar town, Ethiopia. Epidemiology and Health. 2018;**40**:e2018029

[29] Ukke GG, Gurara MK, Boynito WG. Disrespect and abuse of women during childbirth in public health facilities in Arba Minch town, South Ethiopia - a cross-sectional study. PLoS One. 2019;**14**(4):e0205545

[30] Bekele W, Bayou NB, Garedew MG. Magnitude of disrespectful and abusive care among women during facility-based childbirth in Shambu town, Horro Guduru Wollega zone, Ethiopia. Midwifery. 2020;**83**:102629

[31] Adinew YM, Assefa NA. Experience of facility based childbirth in rural

Ethiopia: An exploratory study of Women's perspective. Journal of Pregnancy. 2017;**2017**:7938371

[32] Adinew YM, Hall H, Marshall A, Kelly J. Disrespect and abuse during facility-based childbirth in Central Ethiopia. Global Health Action. 2021;**14**(1):1923327

[33] Bayo P, Belaid L, Tahir EO, Ochola E, Dimiti A, Greco D, et al. "Midwives do not appreciate pregnant women who come to the maternity with torn and dirty clothing": Institutional delivery and postnatal care in Torit County, South Sudan: A mixed method study. BMC Pregnancy and Childbirth. 2020;**20**:1-14

[34] Usso AA, Adem HA, Alemu A, Mohammed A. Disrespect and abuse during childbirth in east Hararghe zone public health facilities, eastern Ethiopia: A cross-sectional study. Frontiers in Global Women's Health. 2023;**4**:1237098

[35] Abuya T, Warren CE, Miller N, Njuki R, Ndwiga C, Maranga A, et al. Exploring the prevalence of disrespect and abuse during childbirth in Kenya. PLoS One. 2015;**10**(4):e0123606

[36] Wassihun B, Zeleke S. Compassionate and respectful maternity care during facility based child birth and women's intent to use maternity service in Bahir Dar, Ethiopia. BMC Pregnancy and Childbirth. 2018;**18**:294

[37] Bulto GA, Demissie DB, Tulu AS. Respectful maternity care during labor and childbirth and associated factors among women who gave birth at health institutions in the west Shewa zone, Oromia region, Central Ethiopia. BMC Pregnancy and Childbirth. 2020;**20**:443

[38] Yosef A, Kebede A, Worku N. Respectful maternity care and associated factors among women who attended delivery services in referral hospitals in Northwest Amhara, Ethiopia: A cross-sectional study. Journal of Multidisciplinary Healthcare Dovepress. 2020;**13**:1965-1973

[39] Amsalu B, Aragaw A, Sintayehu Y, Sema A, Belay Y, Tadese G, et al. Respectful maternity care among laboring women in public hospitals of Benishangul Gumuz region, Ethiopia: A mixed cross-sectional study with direct observations. SAGE Open Medicine. 2022;**10**:20503121221076995

[40] Lagebo BW, Mekonnen SM. Challenges and Approaches to Scaling and Standardizing Health Information Infrastructure in Developing Countries: Case Studies from Ethiopia. Norway: University of Oslo; 2005

[41] Nigusie A, Endehabtu BF, Angaw DA, Teklu A, Mekonnen ZA, Feletto M, et al. Status of compassionate, respectful, and caring health service delivery: Scoping review. JMIR Human Factors. 2022;**9**(1):e30804

Chapter 5

Hope and Scope for Diabetes-Free Generations

V. Seshiah, Anjalakshi Chandrasekar, Pikee Saxena, A. Geetha Lakshmi, N. Bhavatharini and Rajesh Jain

Abstract

Gestational diabetes mellitus (GDM) is a growing global health concern linked to the rising prevalence of obesity and type 2 diabetes. It poses significant short-term and long-term risks for both mothers and their offspring. This comprehensive review explores the concept of early gestational glucose intolerance (EGGI), emphasizing the importance of early detection and intervention to prevent GDM and its adverse outcomes and scope for Diabetes Free Generation. The fuel-mediated teratogenesis hypothesis explains how maternal hyperglycemia disrupts fetal development, leading to macrosomia, neonatal hypoglycemia, and long-term metabolic dysfunction. Early prediction through first-trimester postprandial blood glucose (PPBG) testing allows for timely intervention and management. Recent studies demonstrated the high predictive value of PPBG testing, emphasizing the potential for early identification of women at risk for GDM. Effective management strategies include medical nutrition therapy, exercise, and pharmacological interventions like metformin, particularly when initiated early in pregnancy. The successful intervention program at Chennai and Delhi highlights the efficacy of early detection and proactive management in reducing adverse outcomes. Primordial prevention, focusing on preconception care and early pregnancy screening, is crucial for breaking the cycle of transgenerational transmission of metabolic disorders. By addressing risk factors before and during pregnancy, we can create a healthier future for both mothers and their children. Continued research is needed to validate GDM prevention and management.

Keywords: gestational diabetes mellitus (GDM), early gestational glucose intolerance (EGGI), fuel-mediated teratogenesis, postprandial blood glucose (PPBG), primordial prevention

1. Introduction

Gestational diabetes mellitus (GDM) has emerged as a global health concern, with a steadily increasing prevalence mirroring the rising rates of obesity and type 2 diabetes mellitus (T2DM) in the general population [1]. This alarming trend reflects a broader shift towards sedentary lifestyles and unhealthy dietary patterns, contributing to the growing burden of metabolic disorders worldwide. GDM, defined as glucose intolerance of varying severity with onset or first recognition during pregnancy, not only poses significant risks to maternal and fetal health during pregnancy but also has far-reaching implications for the long-term health of both mother and child [2].

Current understanding of gestational diabetes and in utero fetal programming is based on multifactorial factors (genetic, metabolic, environmental) which include obesity, insulin resistance, inflammation, maternal glucose and lipid metabolism. The complexity of the interactions of these factors provides vast approaches to studying and understanding the maternal, fetal, neonatal, and lifetime effects of gestational diabetes. During pregnancy, hormonal fluctuations, particularly in the second and third trimesters, contribute to increased insulin resistance. This physiological adaptation is essential for ensuring adequate nutrient supply to the developing fetus. However, in women with GDM, this insulin resistance becomes exaggerated, leading to impaired glucose tolerance and hyperglycemia [3]. This metabolic dysregulation creates a cascade of events that can have detrimental effects on both the mother and the fetus, setting the stage for a range of adverse outcomes.

The long-term consequences of GDM extend beyond pregnancy and delivery, casting a shadow over the future health of both mother and child. Women with a history of GDM are at a significantly increased risk of developing T2DM later in life. In fact, GDM is often considered a precursor to T2DM, with a substantial proportion of women progressing to this chronic condition within years or even decades after pregnancy [4]. The offspring of mothers with GDM are also not spared from the adverse effects of this metabolic dysregulation. They are at a higher risk of developing obesity, impaired glucose tolerance, and T2DM in childhood and adulthood, perpetuating a cycle of metabolic dysfunction across generations [5]. This phenomenon, known as "transgenerational transmission" of metabolic disorders, underscores the critical importance of addressing GDM not only as a pregnancy complication but also as a public health issue contributing a major role in the rising prevalence of diabetes with long-lasting implications for future generations.

1.1 The "fuel-mediated teratogenesis" hypothesis

The transgenerational transmission of metabolic dysfunction is intricately linked to the concept of "fuel-mediated teratogenesis." This hypothesis posits that maternal hyperglycemia acts as a teratogenic agent, disrupting normal fetal development and predisposing the offspring to metabolic disorders later in life [6]. In essence, the fetus is exposed to an excess of fuel (mixed nutrients) in utero, which, in turn, triggers a cascade of events that have profound and lasting consequences.

Maternal hyperglycemia leads to increased glucose transfer across the placenta, resulting in fetal hyperglycemia. In response, the fetal pancreas increases insulin production, leading to fetal hyperinsulinemia. Insulin, acting as a growth factor, promotes excessive fetal growth and adiposity, often resulting in macrosomia (a birth weight exceeding 4000 grams) This accelerated growth pattern sets the stage for long-term metabolic dysfunction. The overstimulated fetal beta cells may eventually become exhausted and develop a defective insulin secretory response, contributing to impaired glucose tolerance and insulin resistance in later life [5].

The fuel-mediated teratogenesis hypothesis aligns with the broader concept of developmental origins of health and disease (DOHaD) [7]. This framework emphasizes that environmental exposures during critical periods of fetal development can have a profound and lasting impact on an individual's health trajectory. In the case of GDM, the intrauterine environment, characterized by maternal hyperglycemia, acts as a key programming factor, influencing the development of metabolic systems in the fetus and increasing the risk of metabolic disorders in adulthood. Thus, the concept of fuel-mediated teratogenesis provides a mechanistic explanation for the observed association between GDM and the increased risk of metabolic diseases in offspring, highlighting the importance of maintaining euglycemia during pregnancy to safeguard the health of future generations.

1.2 Problem statement

In light of the far-reaching consequences of GDM for both maternal and fetal health, there is an urgent need to focus on early, prediction, intervention, and prevention strategies to break the cycle of transgenerational transmission of metabolic disorders and pave the way for a diabetes-free generation. In 2018 NIH study suggested that BS screening will identify GDM risk in the first trimester and HbA1c5.3(2 h PPBS>110 mg/dL) in the 10th week predicts GDM.

This chapter aims to provide a comprehensive overview of the current understanding of GDM, and predict and prevent GDM to address this growing global health challenge.

The focus is on the concept of early gestational glucose intolerance (EGGI), a novel approach that emphasizes the detection of glucose intolerance in the first trimester of pregnancy, well before the traditional screening window of 24–28 weeks gestation. This early identification of at-risk women allows for timely intervention and management, potentially preventing the development of GDM and its associated complications. The evidence supporting the efficacy of early intervention strategies, including medical nutrition therapy, exercise, and pharmacological interventions such as metformin, will be explored in detail. Additionally, the chapter will delve into the long-term follow-up of mothers and offspring after GDM, emphasizing the importance of continuous monitoring and preventive measures to mitigate the risk of future metabolic disorders.

The overarching goal of this chapter is to highlight the potential of early detection, intervention, and prevention strategies to break the cycle of transgenerational transmission of metabolic disorders and pave the way for a diabetes-free generation. By focusing on the early stages of pregnancy and implementing comprehensive management approaches, we can strive to improve maternal and fetal health outcomes and reduce the burden of diabetes in future generations.

2. Developmental origins of health and disease

2.1 Embryology of beta cell development

To understand the intricacies of GDM and its impact on fetal development, it is essential to delve into the developmental origins of health and disease, particularly the embryology of beta cell development. The pancreas, a key organ in glucose regulation, undergoes a complex developmental process during fetal life. Pancreatic beta cells, responsible for insulin production, begin to differentiate during the 10th and 11th weeks of gestation and become functionally responsive to glucose levels by the 11th week [8]. This early development highlights the vulnerability of these cells to environmental influences, including maternal glucose levels, during this critical period.

Maternal glucose, the primary fuel for fetal growth, readily crosses the placenta and becomes the main source of energy for the developing fetus. In a normal pregnancy, maternal glucose levels rise after meals, triggering a physiological increase in insulin secretion by the mother. This insulin response helps maintain maternal glycemic control and ensures a steady supply of glucose to the fetus. However, in the presence of GDM, maternal hyperglycemia disrupts this delicate balance. Elevated maternal glucose levels lead to increased glucose transfer across the placenta, resulting in fetal hyperglycemia.

The fetal pancreas, sensing the excess glucose, responds by increasing insulin production. This fetal hyperinsulinemia serves as a compensatory mechanism to promote glucose uptake and utilization by fetal tissues, particularly for growth and energy storage. However, chronic exposure to high glucose levels can have detrimental effects on fetal beta cell function. The overstimulation of beta cells due to persistent hyperglycemia can lead to beta cell exhaustion and dysfunction, impairing their ability to respond adequately to glucose fluctuations in later life [5]. This phenomenon, often referred to as "beta cell exhaustion" is a key factor in the development of insulin resistance and T2DM in offspring exposed to maternal hyperglycemia in utero.

Furthermore, the excess insulin produced by the fetal pancreas acts as a growth factor, promoting accelerated growth of various fetal tissues, including adipose tissue. This accelerated growth can lead to macrosomia, which is associated with an increased risk of birth complications and long-term metabolic consequences for the offspring. Thus, maternal glucose levels play a pivotal role in shaping fetal beta cell development and function (**Figure 1**).

2.2 Intrauterine programming and epigenetics

The detrimental impact of maternal hyperglycemia on fetal beta cell development and function is further exacerbated by the phenomenon of intrauterine programming, also known as fetal programming. This concept refers to the process by which environmental exposures during critical periods of fetal development can induce long-lasting changes in the structure, physiology, and metabolism of the offspring, ultimately influencing their susceptibility to various diseases in later life [7]. In GDM,

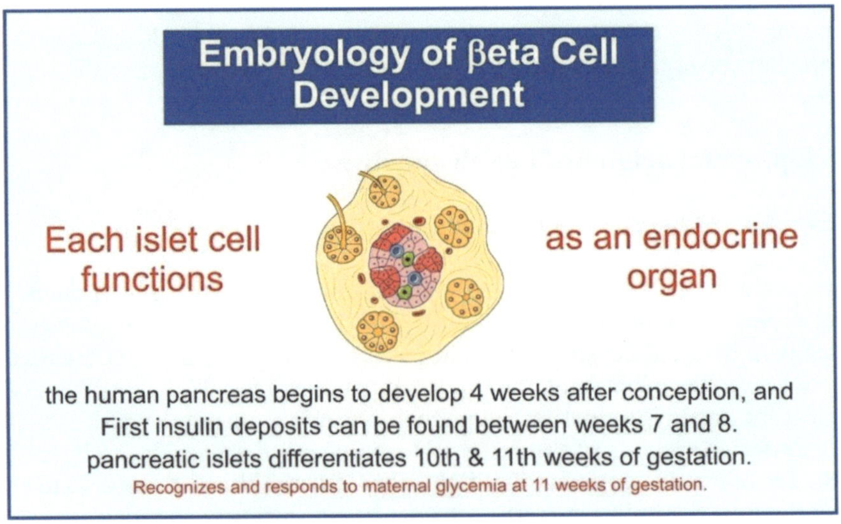

Figure 1.
Cell differentiation during early human development. Credit: V Seshiah.

the intrauterine environment, characterized by maternal hyperglycemia, plays a pivotal role in programming the metabolic fate of the offspring.

Epigenetic mechanisms are central to the process of intrauterine programming. Epigenetics refers to heritable changes in gene expression that occur without alterations to the underlying DNA sequence. These changes are mediated by various mechanisms, including DNA methylation and histone modification. In GDM, maternal hyperglycemia can induce epigenetic modifications in the fetal genome, leading to altered gene expression patterns that persist into adulthood and contribute to the development of metabolic disorders,

DNA methylation, one of the most well-studied epigenetic mechanisms, involves the addition of methyl groups to cytosine residues in DNA. This modification typically results in gene silencing, as methylated DNA is less accessible to transcription factors and other regulatory proteins. Studies have shown that offspring of mothers with GDM exhibit altered DNA methylation patterns in genes involved in glucose metabolism and insulin signaling [9]. These epigenetic changes can disrupt normal metabolic pathways and increase the offspring's susceptibility to insulin resistance, obesity, and T2DM.

Histone modification is another important epigenetic mechanism that plays a crucial role in gene regulation. Histones are proteins around which DNA is wrapped, forming chromatin structures. Modifications of histones, such as acetylation and methylation, can alter chromatin structure and either promote or repress gene expression. Maternal hyperglycemia can induce changes in histone acetylation and methylation patterns in the fetal genome, affecting the expression of genes critical for metabolic regulation and development [3]. These epigenetic changes can persist into adulthood, contributing to the long-term metabolic consequences of GDM (**Figure 2**).

2.3 Fetal origin of adult disease theory

The combined effects of fetal beta cell dysfunction, intrauterine programming, and epigenetic modifications contribute to the fetal origin of adult disease (FOAD)

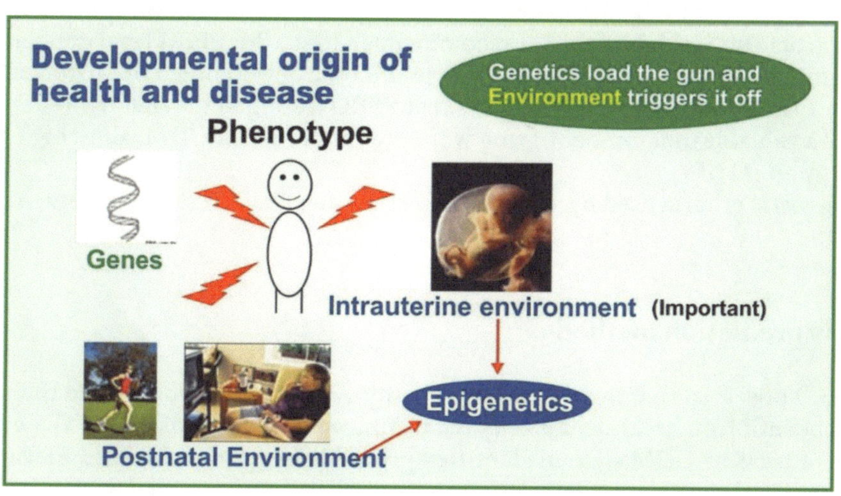

Figure 2.
Intrauterine environment. Credit: Francis Collins.

theory, also known as the developmental origins of health and disease (DOHaD) hypothesis. This theory posits that environmental exposures during fetal development can have a profound and lasting impact on an individual's risk of developing various diseases in adulthood, including metabolic disorders like obesity, T2DM, and cardiovascular disease [7]. In the context of GDM, the FOAD theory highlights the importance of the intrauterine environment in shaping the metabolic health trajectory of the offspring.

The intrauterine exposure to hyperglycemia can have a lasting impact on the offspring's metabolic health, independent of their genetic makeup.

Moreover, the FOAD theory extends beyond glucose metabolism. Studies have shown that offspring of mothers with GDM are also at an increased risk of developing cardiovascular diseases, such as hypertension and dyslipidemia, later in life. This indicates that the adverse effects of maternal hyperglycemia are not limited to glucose homeostasis but can affect multiple physiological systems, contributing to a cluster of metabolic and cardiovascular risk factors in the offspring.

The FOAD theory emphasizes the importance of early intervention to mitigate the long-term consequences of GDM. By identifying and managing GDM early in pregnancy, and potentially breaking the cycle of transgenerational transmission of metabolic disorders and paving the way for a healthier future.

3. Gestational diabetes mellitus: Detection and prediction

The diagnostic test for GDM has gone through many evolutions from two step procedure (ADA) to single test procedure (DIPSI) with various challenges.

The concern is early prediction and intervention which are crucial for mitigating the adverse effects of GDM, especially in populations with limited access to healthcare.

As NIH suggested [10], first-trimester screening allows for the identification of women with early gestational glucose intolerance (EGGI), a condition characterized by elevated postprandial blood glucose (PPBG) levels in the first trimester,

Early identification of EGGI enables timely intervention and management, potentially preventing the progression to GDM and its associated complications. A review article by Seshiah et al. [11] recommended that a 2-h PPBG level greater than 110 mg/dL at 8–10 weeks of gestation can predict the development of GDM with high sensitivity and specificity. This suggests that PPBG testing in the first trimester could serve as a valuable tool for identifying women at high risk for GDM, allowing for early intervention [11].

Diagnostic criteria used by agencies for estimating GDM is shown below in **Table 1**.

4. Early prediction method

W.H.O observed that there is no high quality evidence that women and their fetuses benefit from treatment if only the fasting value is abnormal. RCT shows benefit of treating GDM women identified primarily by post load values. Elevated postprandial plasma glucose may be more predictive of the potential for fetal morbidity compared with fasting plasma glucose. Therefore, fasting glucose values used alone do not predict in the need for pharmacological therapy.

Criteria		Fasting		1-h		2-h		3-h	
		mg/dL	mmol/dL	mg/dL	mmol/dL	mg/dL	mmol/dL	mg/dL	mmol/dL
ADA/ACOG	2003 2018	95	5.3	180	10.0	155	8.6	140	7.8
ADIPS	2014	92	5.1	180	10.0	153	8.5	—	—
Diabetes Canada clinical guidelines	2018	95	5.3	—	10.6	—	9.0	—	—
DIPSI	2014	—	—	—	—	140	7.8	—	—
EASD	1991	110/126	6.1/7.0	—	—	162/180	9.0/100	—	—
FIGO	2015	92	5.1	180	10.0	153	8.5	—	—
WHO	1998	110/126	6.1/7.0	—	—	120/140	6.7/7.8	—	—
WHO	2013	92	5.1	180	10.0	153	8.5	—	—
IADPSG	2010	92	5.1	180	10.0	153	8.5	—	—
NICE	2015	—	5.6	—	—	—	7.8	—	—

Table 1.
Diagnostic criteria used by agencies for estimating GDM.

Based on the hypothesis of EGGI discussed earlier in this paper, a recent study was done including 200 women to evaluate the correlation between first-trimester 2 h postprandial blood glucose (PPBG) ≥ 110 mg/dL for predicting gestational diabetes mellitus. Among women having PPBS ≥ 110 mg/dL, 95.9% developed GDM, while in the group with PPBS < 110 mg/dL, only 4% developed GDM. Women with PPBS ≥ 110 mg/dL had significantly higher rates of cesarean section ($p < 0.01$), preterm delivery ($p < 0.001$), and macrosomia ($p < 0.001$). Area under the curve (AUC) for PPBS was 0.969 ($p < 0.001$) with 95% CI: 0.933–0.988. PPBS ≥ 110 mg/dL has a sensitivity of 95.9%, specificity of 95.6%, positive predictive value (PPV) of 95.9%, negative predictive value (NPV) of 95.7%, and diagnostic accuracy of 95.77% to predict GDM [12]. These findings suggest that PPBG testing in the first trimester could serve as a reliable and practical tool for early GDM prediction.

The advantages of first-trimester PPBG testing are numerous. Early prediction of GDM allows for timely intervention and management, potentially preventing or mitigating the adverse effects of maternal hyperglycemia on both the mother and the fetus. Moreover, PPBG testing is a relatively simple and non-invasive procedure that can be easily integrated into routine prenatal care. PPBG testing can be performed after a standard meal, making it more convenient for both patients and healthcare providers.

The implementation of first-trimester PPBG testing as a routine screening tool has the potential to revolutionize GDM management. By identifying women at high risk for GDM early in pregnancy, healthcare providers can initiate personalized interventions, such as medical nutrition therapy and lifestyle modifications, to optimize glycemic control and reduce the risk of complications. This, proactive approach can lead to improved maternal and fetal outcomes, including a lower risk of macrosomia, preterm birth, and neonatal hypoglycemia.

Gestational diabetes mellitus	PPBS (mg/dL) 2 h at < 12 weeks of POG	HbA1c (%) at < 12 weeks of POG
Area under the ROC curve (AUC)	0.969	0.916
Standard error	0.0145	0.0193
95% confidence interval	0.933–0.988	0.867–0.951
P value	<0.0001	<0.0001
Cut off	≥110 mg/dL	≥5.3%
Sensitivity (95% CI)	95.88% (89.8–98.9%)	81.44% (72.3–88.6%)
Specificity (95% CI)	95.65% (89.2–98.8%)	85.87% (77.0–92.3%)
PPV (95% CI)	95.9% (89.8–98.9%)	85.9% (77.0–92.3%)
NPV (95% CI)	95.7% (89.2–98.8%)	81.4% (72.3–88.6%)
Diagnostic accuracy	95.77%	83.60%

Table 2.
Diagnostic accuracy of PPBS and HbA1c for predicting GDM.

HbA1c, a measure of average blood glucose levels over the past 2–3 months, has been investigated as a potential early predictor of GDM. HbA1c values of ≥6.5% are diagnostic of pre-gestational diabetes and prediabetes prior to pregnancy, is defined as HbA1c between 5.7% and 6.4%. Some studies suggest that an HbA1c level of 5.3% or higher in the first trimester may be associated with an increased risk of developing GDM [10]. However, the use of HbA1c for early GDM screening is still under debate, as its sensitivity and specificity may not be as high as those of PPBG testing [13]. Diagnostic accuracy of PPBS and HbA1c for predicting GDM are shown in **Table 2** [12]. However, larger prospective studies are required to enhance the level of evidence.

The current glycaemic threshold for normoglycemic women during pregnancy has been challenged. Hernandez et al. studied the pattern of glycemia in normal pregnancy by pooling analysis of 12 studies involving 45 years of data. They indicated that the

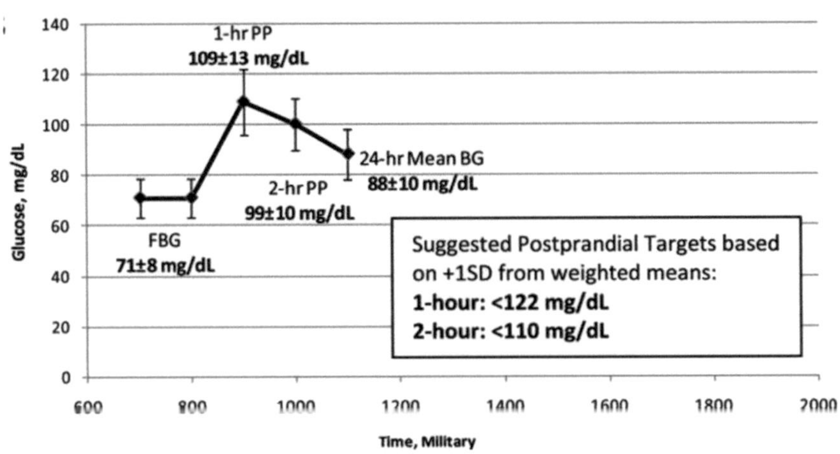

Figure 3.
Patterns of glycemia in normal pregnancy [14]. Credit: Hernandez TL.

glycaemic targets in the management of hyperglycaemia in pregnancy need to be lower than the currently used ones. They detected the normal levels of fasting blood glucose (FBG) to be 71 ± 8 mg/dL (3.9 ± 0.4 mmol/l) and post-prandial blood glucose (PPBG) to be 99 ± 10 mg/dL (5.5 ± 0.6 mmol/l). They have suggested therapeutic PPBG targets of <122 mg/dL (6.8 mmol/l) at 1 h and < 110 mg/dL (6.1 mmol/l) at 2 h (**Figure 3**).

However, prior to making broad antenatal management recommendations, larger prospective studies are required to enhance the level of evidence.

5. Prevention and management strategies

Early intervention, ideally before 11 weeks of gestation, aims to normalize maternal glucose levels and prevent fetal hyperinsulinemia. By intervening early, we can potentially protect the developing beta cells from the detrimental effects of excess glucose and insulin, thus reducing the risk of long-term metabolic dysfunction in the offspring. This approach aligns with the concept of "metabolic memory," which suggests that early exposure to hyperglycemia can have lasting effects on metabolic health, even after glucose levels are normalized [9]. In other words, the metabolic milieu experienced during fetal development can leave a lasting imprint on the individual's metabolic programming, influencing their risk of developing metabolic disorders later in life.

The concept of metabolic memory emphasizes the importance of early intervention in GDM, as it suggests that the prevention of hyperglycemia in the early stages of pregnancy can have long-lasting benefits for both mother and child. By maintaining optimal glycemic control from the outset, we can potentially alter the course of fetal development and reduce the risk of adverse metabolic programming. This proactive approach has the potential to break the cycle of transgenerational transmission of metabolic disorders and create a healthier future for generations to come.

The cornerstone of early intervention in GDM lies in the implementation of effective management strategies, with medical nutrition therapy (MNT) and exercise playing a pivotal role. MNT involves personalized dietary counseling and education aimed at optimizing glycemic control while ensuring adequate nutrition for both the mother and the developing fetus.

Specific dietary recommendations for women with GDM include distributing carbohydrate intake throughout the day to avoid large spikes in blood glucose levels. This typically involves consuming three smalls to moderate-sized meals and two to three snacks daily, with a focus on complex carbohydrates with a low glycemic index [14]. Low glycemic index foods, such as whole grains, legumes, and vegetables, are digested more slowly and release glucose into the bloodstream gradually, preventing rapid fluctuations in blood sugar levels.

The total carbohydrate intake is usually restricted to 50% of total daily calories, with an emphasis on fiber-rich sources that promote satiety and slow down glucose absorption. Protein intake is recommended to be around 20–25% of total calories, while fat should comprise 20–25% of total calories, prioritizing healthy fats like those found in nuts, seeds, and olive oil.

In addition to carbohydrate distribution, meal timing is crucial for glycemic control in women with GDM. Consuming a small breakfast is often recommended, as insulin resistance tends to be highest in the morning. Spacing meals and snacks evenly throughout the day helps maintain stable blood glucose levels and prevents prolonged periods of fasting, which can lead to increased hepatic glucose production and elevated fasting glucose levels.

5.1 Pharmacological interventions

While MNT and exercise are the first-line interventions for EGGI, pharmacological therapy may be necessary in cases where lifestyle modifications alone are insufficient to achieve optimal glycemic control. Pharmacotherapy in the form of Insulin or oral antidiabetic agent like Metformin may be required to bring down PPBG levels below 110 mg/dL within a short period of 1–2 weeks for preventing intrauterine programming by 10 weeks. Efficacy and safety of insulin is already well established as it does not cross the placental barrier and it is regarded as the first line therapy for managing hyperglycemia. The dose of insulin can be titrated according to the level of hyperglycemia and the onset and duration of action can be modified by using different preparations alone or in combination. Besides conventional Regular and NPH insulin, rapid insulin analogues like Aspart and Lispro, long acting basal insulin, like Detemir, Degludec and Glargine have been approved for use during pregnancy. Although such a wide variety of insulin are available, majority of the pregnant women are scared or not willing to use insulin in the real life situation. The requirement of repeated injections, regular monitoring of plasma glucose levels, risk of hypoglycemia, higher cost and need for refrigeration, taboo of insulin therapy and labeling as a diabetic patient are some of the deterrents for use of insulin during pregnancy.

Metformin, an oral biguanide medication, has emerged as a safe and effective option for managing GDM, particularly in women with EGGI or those who require additional support to achieve glycemic targets. The advantages of Metformin over insulin therapy are it's oral administration, low cost, easy availability, no need for refrigeration, minimum risk of hypoglycemia, it does not require very strict glucose monitoring and evidence of it's safety and efficacy over the years make it the popular choice for the clinicians and the pregnant women. Moreover, the obstetricians have the experience of using Metformin for women with PCOS and have continued it during pregnancy. Most obstetricians are not comfortable to recommend insulin therapy for pregnant women. Therefore, for the masses, Metformin therapy appears to be the rational approach.

Extensive research supports the safety and efficacy of metformin in pregnancy. Multiple studies have demonstrated that metformin does not increase the risk of congenital anomalies or adverse neonatal outcomes [15]. Furthermore, metformin has been shown to effectively reduce maternal fasting and postprandial glucose levels, leading to improved glycemic control and a decreased risk of complications such as macrosomia and preeclampsia, the mechanism of action of metformin involves reducing hepatic glucose production, improving insulin sensitivity, and increasing glucose uptake by peripheral tissues. It does not stimulate insulin secretion, thereby minimizing the risk of hypoglycemia.

Regarding the optimal timing for metformin initiation, the emerging evidence suggests that earlier intervention may be more beneficial. Given that fetal beta cells begin secreting insulin around the 11th week of gestation, initiating metformin treatment before this critical period may be crucial for preventing fetal hyperinsulinemia and its associated adverse effects. As discussed earlier, a previous study by Saxena et al [12] has proven that amongst women with EGGI having PPBS > 110 mg/dL, 95.9% developed GDM, while in the group with PPBS < 110 mg/dL, only 4% developed GDM. Based on this study, a recent study by Seshiah et al. [16] demonstrated that metformin administration in women with EGGI, starting at 8 weeks' gestation, effectively maintained postprandial blood glucose levels below 110 mg/dL, only 1 out of 69 (1.4%)

Outcome	N = 70 PPBS>=110 mg/dl EGGI group Metformin Mean ± SDNo.(%)	N = 82 PPBS<110 mg/dl Normoglycemic group No intervention Mean ± SDNo.(%)	P-value
Primary pregnancy outcomes			
PPBS – 8 weeks	111.6 ± 6.2	97.6 ± 6.8	0.000
PPBS – 9 weeks	109.3 ± 6.6	97.6 ± 6.5	0.000
PPBS – 10 weeks	107.1 ± 4.7	97.3 ± 7.0	0.000
PPBS – 11 weeks	105.8 ± 3.8	97.2 ± 7.7	0.000
OGCT – 16 weeks	110.2 ± 12.0	108.3 ± 11.9	0.353
OGCT – 24 weeks	112.4 ± 11.7	109.1 ± 14.6	0.133
OGCT – 32 weeks	110.8 ± 10.8	110.8 ± 7.9	0.976
Birth weight (kg.)	3.0 ± 0.4	2.9 ± 0.4	0.360
<2.5 kg	8(11.4)	10(13.7)	
≥3.5	6 (8.5)	9(12.3)	
LSCS	17 (24.2)	21 (23.6)	0.633
Vaginal delivery	52(74.2)	61(74.4)	

Table 3.
Postprandial glucose levels and pregnancy outcomes in women with early gestational glucose tolerance (EGGI) and normoglycemic women.

women developed GDM and the adverse neonatal outcomes were also similar to the normoglycaemic group (**Table 3**).

The early initiation of metformin, particularly in women with EGGI or those at high risk of developing GDM, aligns with the concept of primordial prevention. By intervening before the onset of significant hyperglycemia and fetal hyperinsulinemia, we can potentially alter the course of fetal development and reduce the risk of long-term metabolic dysfunction in the offspring.

Metformin is generally considered safe during pregnancy; further research is needed to fully elucidate its long-term effects on both the mother and the offspring.

6. Case study from Chennai: Intervention program

The Madras Medical College, India, implemented a successful intervention program to address EGGI in pregnant women [16]. The program focused on maintaining optimal glycemic control and improving maternal and fetal outcomes. Women were enrolled in the study at 8 weeks. Pregnant women with PPBG levels exceeding 110 mg/dL were identified as at risk for developing GDM, and they were included in the intervention group. Non-intervention group included women at 8 weeks gestation having PPBG below 110 mg/dL. Weekly blood sugar trends were followed at 8, 9, 10, 11, 16, 24 and 32 weeks gestation.

The intervention program included medical nutrition therapy (MNT), exercise recommendations, and metformin administration. The MNT component emphasized a balanced diet tailored to meet pregnancy nutritional needs while keeping blood glucose levels stable. This involved distributing carbohydrate intake throughout the day, focusing on complex carbohydrates with a low glycemic index, and ensuring adequate protein and healthy fat intake. The goal was to achieve and maintain postprandial blood glucose levels below 110 mg/dL, thereby reducing the risk of adverse outcomes for both mother and child [12].

Exercise was also an integral part of the intervention, as physical activity has been shown to improve insulin sensitivity and glycemic control. Women were encouraged to engage in moderate-intensity aerobic activities for at least 150 min per week. The results of the intervention program were promising, with blood glucose levels remained significantly lower in the intervention group.

Among the 70 women in the intervention group, blood glucose levels remained significantly lower throughout the early weeks of pregnancy. For instance, the mean PPBG levels at 8 weeks were 111.6 mg/dL in the intervention group compared to 97.6 mg/dL in the euglycaemic group, with a statistically significant difference ($p < 0.000$) (**Figure 4**). By the 11th week, the intervention group continued to show lower glucose levels, demonstrating the effectiveness of the early intervention in maintaining glycemic control and thus prevented intrauterine programming.

The program's impact extended beyond glycemic control to include significant reductions in adverse neonatal outcomes. The composite adverse outcomes, including preterm delivery, large for gestational age (LGA) infants, and the need for neonatal interventions such as phototherapy, were notably lower in the intervention group. Demonstrating the importance of early detection and proactive management in preventing complications associated with GDM.

The intervention program also aimed to establish a framework for long-term health. Women with a history of GDM are at increased risk for developing type 2 diabetes mellitus (T2DM) later in life, and the program included education on lifestyle modifications to reduce this risk. Participants received guidance on maintaining a healthy diet and engaging in regular physical activity postpartum, emphasizing the importance of ongoing health management beyond pregnancy.

The success of this intervention program serves as a model for future GDM management strategies, emphasizing the critical importance of addressing GDM proactively to mitigate immediate risks and promote long-term health. Thus, there is" Hope and Scope" for prevention of diabetes.

7. Future directions

The success of the Madras Medical College intervention program, as evidenced by the significant reduction in blood glucose levels and adverse neonatal outcomes in the intervention group, highlights the potential of early detection and proactive management in mitigating the impact of GDM. Although this study had a small sample size and further, adequately powered studies are required to generate robust date to include it in future guidelines. However, this success story serves as a model for future GDM management strategies, emphasizing the critical importance of addressing GDM at its earliest stages (stage of EGGI) to promote optimal maternal and fetal health. However, to truly break the cycle of transgenerational transmission of metabolic disorders and achieve a diabetes-free generation, we must shift our focus from intervention to prevention, embracing the concept of primordial prevention.

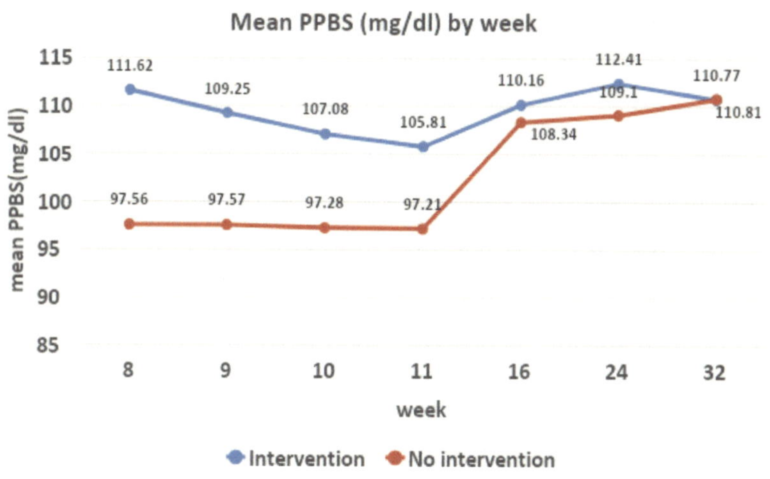

Figure 4.
Mean glycemic level (mg/dL) by weeks in the two groups.

Preconception care and early pregnancy screening are essential components of primordial prevention in GDM. Preconception care involves optimizing a woman's health before pregnancy, addressing modifiable risk factors such as obesity, physical inactivity, and poor nutrition. By promoting healthy lifestyle habits and addressing underlying health conditions before conception, we can create a favorable intrauterine environment for the developing fetus and reduce the risk of GDM.

Early pregnancy screening, particularly in the first trimester, allows for the timely identification of women at risk for GDM. The use of first-trimester PPBG testing, as demonstrated in the Delhi study, can accurately predict the development of GDM, enabling early intervention and management to prevent complications.

7.1 Use of CGMS

Continuous glucose monitoring (CGM) technology is also emerging as a valuable tool for early GDM detection and management. This allows for a more comprehensive understanding of glycemic patterns and variability, potentially identifying women with subtle glucose intolerance that may not be detected by traditional intermittent testing [17]. Studies have shown that CGM can improve glycemic control in women with GDM, potentially reducing the risk of complications for both mother and child.

7.2 Novel biomarkers

They could potentially predict GDM earlier in pregnancy. These include microRNAs, small non-coding RNA molecules that regulate gene expression, and inflammatory markers, such as C-reactive protein and interleukin-6, which are elevated in women with GDM [9]. The identification of reliable biomarkers could lead to the development of more accurate and personalized risk assessment tools for GDM, enabling targeted interventions for women at highest risk.

The importance of focusing on the female gender in diabetes prevention cannot be overstated. Women play a crucial role in the transgenerational transmission of metabolic disorders, as their health during pregnancy directly influences the health of their offspring. By prioritizing women's health and implementing primordial prevention strategies, we can break this cycle and create a healthier future for generations to come.

7.3 Conclusion

While preconception care and early pregnancy screening are important pillars of primordial prevention, research is ongoing to identify additional avenues for intervention. This includes the investigation of novel biomarkers that can predict GDM risk even before pregnancy, as well as the development of targeted lifestyle interventions that can be implemented at the community level to promote healthy behaviors and reduce the prevalence of obesity and metabolic dysfunction. Future studies should also focus on evaluating the long-term impact of early GDM detection and intervention on the health of offspring, tracking their metabolic and cardiovascular health throughout childhood and adulthood.

In conclusion, GDM is a complex and multifaceted condition with significant implications for both maternal and fetal health. The increasing prevalence of GDM worldwide necessitates a paradigm shift in our approach to its management, focusing on early prediction, intervention, and prevention. The concept of EGGI, with its emphasis on first-trimester PPBG testing, offers a promising avenue for identifying women at risk and initiating timely interventions. By combining early prediction with comprehensive management strategies, including MNT, exercise, and pharmacological therapy, we can strive to optimize glycemic control during pregnancy and reduce the risk of adverse outcomes.

Furthermore, the concept of primordial prevention, with its focus on preconception care and early pregnancy screening, holds the key to breaking the cycle of transgenerational transmission of metabolic disorders. By addressing risk factors before conception and intervening early in pregnancy, we can create a healthier environment for the developing fetus and reduce the long-term burden of metabolic disease. The journey towards a diabetes-free generation requires a concerted effort from healthcare providers, researchers, policymakers, and individuals alike. By prioritizing women's health and implementing evidence-based strategies for GDM prevention and management, we can pave the way for a brighter and healthier future for all with a diabetic free generations.

DOI: http://dx.doi.org/10.5772/intechopen.1007448

Author details

V. Seshiah[1*], Anjalakshi Chandrasekar[2], Pikee Saxena[3], A. Geetha Lakshmi[4], N. Bhavatharini[5] and Rajesh Jain[6]

1 Tamil Nadu Dr. MGR Medical University, Chennai, India

2 Obstetrics and Gynecology, Madras Medical College and Research Institute, Chennai, India

3 Obstetrics and Gynecology, Lady Hardinge Medical College and Associated Hospitals, New Delhi, India

4 Obstetrics and Gynecology, Madras Medical College, Chennai, India

5 SRC Diabetes Centre, Erode, India

6 Jain Hospital and Research Centre, Kanpur, India

*Address all correspondence to: vseshiah@gmail.com

References

[1] Mokdad AH, Ford ES, Bowman BA, Dietz WH, Vinicor F, Bales VS, et al. Prevalence of obesity, diabetes, and obesity-related health risk factors. JAMA. 2001;**289**(1):76-79. DOI: 10.1001/jama.289.1.76

[2] Seshiah V, Balaji V, Balaji MS, Sanjeevi CB, Green A. Gestational diabetes mellitus in India. The Journal of the Association of Physicians of India. 2004;**52**:707-711

[3] Desoye G, Nolan CJ. The fetal glucose steal: An underappreciated phenomenon in diabetic pregnancy. Diabetologia. 2016;**59**(6):1089-1094. DOI: 10.1007/s00125-016-3931-6

[4] Dornhorst A, Rossi M. Risk and prevention of type 2 diabetes in women with gestational diabetes. Diabetes Care. 1998;**21**(Suppl. 2):B43-B49

[5] Sobngwi E, Boudou P, Mauvais-Jarvis F, et al. Effect of a diabetic environment in utero on predisposition to type 2 diabetes. Lancet. 2003;**361**:1861-1865. DOI: 10.1016/S0140-6736(03)13505-2

[6] Freinkel N. Banting Lecture 1980. Of pregnancy and progeny. Diabetes. 1980;**29**(12):1023-1035. DOI: 10.2337/diab.29.12.1023

[7] Barker DJP. The fetal and infant origins of adult disease. British Medical Journal. 1990;**301**(6761):1111. DOI: 10.1136/bmj.301.6761.1111

[8] Piper K, Brickwood S, Turnpenny LW, Cameron IT, Ball SG, Wilson DI, et al. Beta cell differentiation during early human pancreas development. Journal of Endocrinology. 2004;**181**(1):11-23. DOI: 10.1677/joe.0.1810011

[9] Goyal D, Limesand SW, Goyal R. Epigenetic responses and the developmental origins of health and disease. The Journal of Endocrinology. 2019;**242**(1):T105-T119. DOI: 10.1530/JOE-19-0009

[10] American Diabetes Association. 2. Classification and diagnosis of diabetes: Standards of medical care in diabetes—2020. Diabetes Care. 2020;**43**(Supplement 1):S14-S31. DOI: 10.2337/dc20-S002

[11] Seshiah V, Bronson SC, Balaji V, Jain R, Anjalakshi C. Prediction and prevention of gestational diabetes mellitus and its sequelae by administering metformin in the early weeks of pregnancy. Cureus. 2022;**14**(11):e31532. DOI: 10.7759/cureus.31532

[12] Saxena P, Yadav A, Singh M, et al. Correlation between the first trimester two-hour postprandial blood glucose greater than 110 mg/dL for the prediction of gestational diabetes mellitus. Cureus. 2024;**16**(8):e66652. DOI: 10.7759/cureus.66652

[13] Hinkle SN, Tsai MY, Rawal S, Albert PS, Zhang C. HbA_{1c} measured in the first trimester of pregnancy and the association with gestational diabetes. Scientific Reports. 2018;**8**(1):12249. DOI: 10.1038/s41598-018-30833-8

[14] Hernandez TL, Friedman JE, Van Pelt RE, Barbour LA. Patterns of glycemia in normal pregnancy: Should the current therapeutic targets be challenged? Diabetes Care. 2011;**34**:1660-1668. DOI: 10.2337/dc11-0241

[15] Brand KMG, Saarelainen L, Sonajalg J, Boutmy E, et al. Metformin

in pregnancy and risk of adverse long-term outcomes: A register-based cohort study. BMJ Open Diabetes Research & Care. 2022;**10**(1):e002363. DOI: 10.1136/bmjdrc-2021-002363

[16] Veerasamy S, Balaji V, Chawla R, Sahay R, Divakar H, Das AK, et al. DIPSI 2024 — Delhi declaration — A futuristic approach towards primordial prevention of diabetes. International Journal of Diabetes in Developing Countries. 2024;**44**(Suppl 1):S53-S601. DOI: 10.1007/s13410-023-01236-x

[17] Liang X, Fu Y, Lu S, Shuai M, Miao Z, et al. Continuous glucose monitoring-derived glycemic metrics and adverse pregnancy outcomes among women with gestational diabetes: A prospective cohort study. The LANCET Regional Health Western Pacific. 2023;**39**:100823. DOI: 10.1016/j.lanwpc.2023.100823

Section 2

Clinical Care, Interventions, and Delivery Outcomes

Chapter 6

Labor and Delivery Care: The Four Stages

Fatemeh Ahadi Yulghunlu

Abstract

In labor and delivery care, we need to have a single and broad view of the total process of labor, delivery, and neonate birth. Key considerations during labor include the four "P's": power, pass, passenger, and psyche. These elements are vital for assessing the effectiveness of contractions, the passage through the birth canal, and the condition of the fetus, respectively. Continuous monitoring of the fetal heart rate is also crucial to ensuring the well-being of the unborn child throughout the labor process. Also, in delivery care, recognizing the time of completion of the second stage and preparing the mother for pushing and paying attention to the descent of the fetus and the need to perform an episiotomy and finally the birth of the neonate. All these steps require a systematic approach, and it is predetermined that we know the normal process to recognize the abnormal cases and take the correct action.

Keywords: midwifery care, labor care, delivery care, progress of labor, fetal monitoring

1. Introduction

Labor and delivery care is a critical aspect of maternal health, encompassing the processes and practices involved in supporting women through childbirth. This period is marked by significant physiological and emotional changes, requiring comprehensive and compassionate care to ensure the well-being of both the mother and the newborn [1].

The labor journey begins with the onset of regular contractions, leading to the dilation and effacement of the cervix. This process is divided into four stages: the first stage involves early and active labor, the second stage culminates in the delivery of the baby, the third stage concludes with the delivery of the placenta, and the fourth stage is the first two hours after delivery, which is called recovery [1, 2].

Each stage presents unique challenges and requires specific interventions to manage pain, monitor fetal well-being, and address any complications that may arise.

Effective labor and delivery care is grounded in evidence-based practices that prioritize safety, minimize unnecessary interventions, and promote a positive birth experience. Healthcare providers, including obstetricians, midwives, and nurses, are pivotal in offering continuous support, education, and medical care to mothers [3].

Knowing the processes of the labor period (the period with labor pains), the needs of the mother and her care, as well as the birth process, the way of delivery, and the necessary interventions enable health professionals, especially midwives, who are the standard of birth attendants, to guide and manage labor and delivery well and perform the necessary interventions at the right time, so that the mother and her fetus can finish this period with the least complications [4].

Labor has four stages that start with labor pains and finally end with delivery. Now, in this chapter, these necessary steps and interventions are explained.

Ultimately, labor and delivery care is a testament to the dedication and expertise of healthcare professionals, ensuring that every mother and newborn receives the highest standard of care during one of life's most transformative moments.

2. The first stage of labor

Labor is defined by intense and painful uterine contractions that facilitate cervical dilation and enable the descent of the fetus through the birth canal. However, significant preparatory processes occur in both the uterus and cervix well in advance of this stage. Throughout the initial 36–38 weeks of a typical gestation period, the myometrium remains in a preparatory state, characterized by unresponsiveness. Simultaneously, the cervix initiates an early remodeling phase while preserving its structural integrity. Following this period of uterine quiescence, a transitional phase commences, during which the myometrium's unresponsiveness is temporarily lifted and the cervix undergoes processes of ripening, effacement, and a reduction in structural cohesion [5].

The first stage of childbirth includes two phases:

2.1 Early labor

Early labor, also known as the latent phase, is the initial part of the first stage. During this phase, the relaxation of the uterus is disrupted, the cervix becomes soft, and the receptors in the myometrium wall of the uterus respond to uterotonics. Then contractions begin to occur at regular intervals, although they are usually mild and may not be very painful. The cervix starts to soften, thin out (efface), and dilate up to 6 centimeters. This phase can last for several hours to days, especially for first-time mothers [6].

During early labor, it is common for women to experience a range of symptoms, including:

- Mild to moderate contractions that may feel like menstrual cramps.
- A clear or slightly bloody discharge from the vagina, known as the mucus plug.
- Backache or a sensation of pressure in the lower abdomen.

To manage discomfort during early labor, women are encouraged to stay active, practice relaxation techniques, and stay hydrated. Many women spend this phase at home until contractions become more intense and frequent [7].

The following strategies may be effective in managing labor pains and associated discomfort:

- Engage in a cycle of rest and ambulation: It is advisable to alternate between periods of rest and movement while also experimenting with various positions to alleviate discomfort.

- Practice slow, deep breathing techniques: It is important to remain relaxed during contractions; therefore, focus on breathing through each contraction to the best of your ability.

- Maintain adequate hydration: Ensure that you are consuming sufficient fluids and consult with your healthcare provider regarding the appropriateness of light eating or the necessity of fasting during this period [8].

- Consider engaging in hydrotherapy, as activities such as bathing, showering, or swimming in a pool may provide relief. It is advisable to consult with your healthcare provider before undertaking these activities, particularly if your amniotic membranes have ruptured.

- Additionally, prioritize self-care by utilizing aromatherapy, music, and your support network to facilitate positive distractions [9].

2.2 Active labor

Active labor is the second phase of the first stage and is marked by more intense and frequent contractions. During this phase, the cervix dilates from 6 to 10 centimeters. Contractions become stronger, closer together, and more regular. This phase is typically shorter than early labor but can still last several hours [10].

As active labor progresses, women may experience:

- Stronger and more painful contractions.

- Increased pressure in the lower back and pelvis.

- Possible rupture of the amniotic sac (water breaking).

It is usually recommended to go to the hospital or birthing center during active labor. Healthcare providers will monitor the mother and baby closely, providing support and pain relief as needed [11].

2.3 Midwifery care

This section documents the woman's name along with essential information necessary for assessing her baseline characteristics and risk status upon admission for labor. Additionally, pertinent demographic and labor-related factors, including the woman's age, gestational age, serological results, hemoglobin levels, blood type and Rh factor, referral status and rationale, and symphysis-fundal height, should be incorporated into the woman's medical record [3].

Table 1 shows how to assess the variables discussed in this section, as well as the appropriate manner for documenting the acquired information [3].

Variable	Step 1: Assess	Step 2: Record
Name	Ask the woman her full name.	• Record the woman's full name and verify that it matches the name on her medical record.
Parity	Extract from medical records the number of times the woman has given birth to a baby after the age of viability (as per local guidelines).	• Use the local coding system to record parity, e.g., Parity (or P) = number of babies born (after the local definition of viability).
Labor onset	Was the onset of labor spontaneous or induced (using any artificial means)?	• Record "Spontaneous" if the woman achieved the active first stage of labor without any artificial stimulation of labor onset (either through pharmacological or nonpharmacological means). • Record "Induced" if the onset of labor was artificially stimulated by administering oxytocin or prostaglandins to the pregnant woman, artificially rupturing the amniotic membranes, applying a balloon catheter into the cervix, or any other means.
Active labor diagnosis	On what date was the active first stage of labor diagnosed?	• Date of active labor diagnosis. Use local format to record dates (e.g., dd/mm/yy, mm/dd/yy, or dd/ mm/yyyy).
Ruptured membranes	On what date and at what time were amniotic membranes ruptured (if membranes have ruptured before admission)?	• Date and time [hh: mm] that rupture of membranes occurred. These data could be reported by the woman or her companion, or they could be extracted from medical records if membranes ruptured after admission but before initiating the LCG. • Use local format to record time. • Record "U" or "unknown" if rupture of membranes is confirmed and the woman cannot report the date and/ or time and there is no documentation in the medical record.
Risk factor	Risk factors	• Known obstetric, medical, and social risk factors with implications for care provision and potential outcome of labor management. For example, preexisting medical conditions (e.g., chronic hypertension), obstetric conditions (e.g., pre-eclampsia), woman's advanced age, adolescent pregnancy, preterm labor, and group B Streptococcus colonization.

***Table 1** is modified from WHO Labor Care Guide User's Manual Copyright 2020.*
LCG: labor care guide.

Table 1.
Guidance for completing Section 1.

2.4 Special considerations in the first stage of childbirth include

2.4.1 Control of labor pains

2.4.1.1 Nonmedical methods

1. Breathing techniques: Practicing deep, rhythmic breathing can help manage pain and keep calm. Studies have shown that controlled breathing can reduce the perception of pain and anxiety during labor [12].

2. Movement and positioning: Changing positions, walking, or swaying can help ease discomfort and speed up labor. Research indicates that upright positions and movement can reduce the duration of labor and the need for pain relief [12].

3. Water therapy: Taking a warm bath or shower can relax muscles and reduce pain. Hydrotherapy has been found to decrease pain intensity and improve satisfaction with the childbirth experience [13].

4. Massage and counter pressure: Having a partner or doula apply pressure to your lower back or massage tense areas can provide significant relief. Evidence suggests that massage can reduce labor pain and anxiety [14].

2.4.1.2 Medical methods

1. Epidural analgesia: This is a common and effective method for pain relief during labor. It involves injecting anesthetic near the spinal cord to block pain. Studies show that epidurals provide significant pain relief and are safe for both mother and baby [15].

2. Nitrous oxide: Also known as laughing gas, this can be inhaled during contractions to reduce pain and anxiety. Research supports its effectiveness and safety for pain management during labor [16].

3. Opioids: These can be administered through an IV or injection to help manage severe pain. While effective, they can have side effects and are typically used when other methods are insufficient [17].

2.4.1.3 Psychological support

1. Continuous labor support: Having a doula or continuous support person can significantly reduce the need for pain relief and improve overall birth outcomes [18].

2. Hypnobirthing: This involves using hypnosis techniques to manage pain and anxiety. Studies have shown that hypnobirthing can reduce the need for medical pain relief and improve the childbirth experience [19, 20].

2.4.2 Checking the progress of labor

Monitoring the progress of labor is essential to ensuring the health and safety of both the mother and the baby. Here are some key methods used to check labor progress:

2.4.2.1 Cervical dilation and effacement

- Cervical dilation: Cervical dilatation speed is 1.2 cm per hour in nulliparous women and 1.5 cm per hour in multiparous women. In case of prolongation or arrest of dilatation, the causes, such as sero-pelvic disproportion (CPD), should be investigated [1].

- Effacement: This refers to the thinning of the cervix, measured in percentages from 0–100%. Complete effacement (100%) means the cervix is fully thinned out [1].

2.4.2.2 Contraction monitoring frequency and duration

The frequency, duration, and intensity of contractions are monitored to assess labor progress. Regular, strong contractions that increase in frequency and duration indicate active labor [21].

2.4.2.3 Fetal descent station

This measures the position of the baby's head about the mother's pelvis, ranging from −3 (high in the pelvis) to +3 (crowning). A positive station indicates the baby is moving down the birth canal [22].

2.4.2.4 Vaginal examinations

Manual checks: Midwives perform vaginal examinations to assess cervical dilation, effacement, and the baby's position. These checks are crucial for determining the stage of labor [23].

2.4.2.5 Use of partogram

Graphical tool: A partogram is a chart used to plot the progress of labor, including cervical dilation, fetal heart rate, and contraction patterns. It helps in identifying any deviations from the normal labor progression [24].

2.4.2.6 Ultrasound and sonographic assessment

Imaging techniques: Ultrasound can be used to assess fetal position, amniotic fluid levels, and other factors that might affect labor progress. It provides a noninvasive way to monitor labor [25].

2.4.2.7 Maternal vital signs

Monitoring health: Checking the mother's blood pressure, pulse, and temperature helps ensure her well-being during labor. Abnormal vital signs can indicate complications [1].

In general, the four Ps are important in checking the progress of labor, which include four Ps (power, passenger, passage, and psyche).

Labor progress is determined by assessing the four following components, also known as the four Ps:

1. Power: The term "power" pertains to the intensity of uterine contractions and the maternal efforts to expel the fetus during the second stage of labor. This aspect is evaluated through abdominal palpation. Contractions that contribute to normal labor progression should exhibit regularity, frequency, a duration exceeding 60 seconds, and facilitate cervical effacement.

2. Passenger: This pertains to the evaluation of the fetus, specifically regarding its size, position, and attitude, which refers to the spatial relationship among the

various fetal parts. Additionally, it is essential to be cognizant of any underlying conditions that may raise concerns regarding the progress of the pregnancy [24].

3. Passage: The anatomy of the bony pelvis must be evaluated in conjunction with soft tissue elements, including the existence of a distended bladder or rectum, any occupying masses, or the presence of vaginal septa. The assessment of pelvic adequacy can only be conducted during the process of labor.

4. Psyche: This analysis acknowledges the significance of the mother's emotional state during labor, which can influence the overall progression of the labor process. Key factors to evaluate include the levels of stress and underlying anxiety experienced by the mother, the presence of sufficient support from a birthing partner, and the establishment of a welcoming and supportive environment for the woman [24].

In the **Figure 1**, the Friedman curve shows the progress of labor [26].

2.5 Check and monitor fetal heart rate

Monitoring the fetal heart rate (FHR) during labor is crucial for assessing the baby's well-being and ensuring a safe delivery. Here are the key methods and their importance [27].

1. Auscultation: This involves periodically listening to the fetal heartbeat using a special stethoscope or a Doppler device. It helps detect any irregularities in the heart rate that might indicate fetal distress [28].

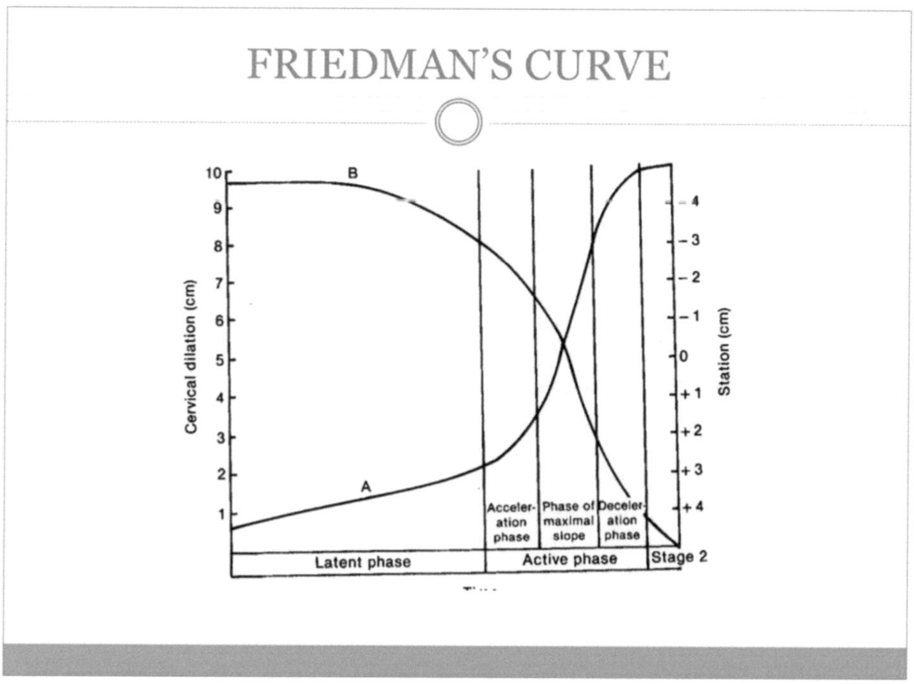

Figure 1.
Friedman curve diagram.

2. Electronic fetal monitoring (EFM): EFM uses external or internal devices to continuously record the fetal heart rate and uterine contractions.

    - External monitoring: Involves placing two belts around the mother's abdomen. One belt uses Doppler ultrasound to detect the fetal heart rate, while the other measures contractions.

    - Internal monitoring: Involves inserting a small electrode through the cervix and attaching it to the baby's scalp to directly measure the heart rate. Provides a continuous record of the fetal heart rate, allowing for real-time assessment and immediate intervention if needed [29].

2.6 Mother's emotional needs

Addressing the emotional needs of mothers during labor is crucial for a positive childbirth experience. Here are some key aspects to consider:

1. Emotional support

    - Continuous presence: Having a continuous support person, such as a partner, doula, or nurse, can significantly reduce anxiety and stress. Continuous support has been shown to improve birth outcomes and increase maternal satisfaction [30].

    - Encouragement and reassurance: Providing words of encouragement and reassurance helps mothers feel more confident and in control during labor [31].

2. Respect and dignity

    - Respectful care: Ensuring that the mother is treated with respect and dignity throughout labor is essential. This includes maintaining her privacy, obtaining informed consent, and respecting her birth plan [32].

    - Cultural sensitivity: Being aware of and respecting cultural practices and preferences can help mothers feel more comfortable and supported [32].

3. Information and communication

    - Clear communication: Keeping the mother informed about the progress of labor and any procedures being performed helps reduce fear and uncertainty [33].

    - Informed decision-making: Encouraging the mother to ask questions and participate in decision-making empowers her and enhances her sense of control [34].

4. Physical comfort

    - Comfort measures: Providing physical comfort measures, such as pillows, warm blankets, and a comfortable environment, can help mothers feel more at ease.

- Mobility and positioning: Allowing the mother to move around and choose comfortable positions during labor can help reduce discomfort and improve labor progress.

5. Psychological support

- Addressing fears and anxieties: Acknowledging and addressing any fears or anxieties the mother may have about labor and childbirth is crucial for her emotional well-being.

- Positive birth environment: Creating a calm and supportive birth environment can help reduce stress and promote a positive birth experience [31].

Meeting the emotional needs of mothers during labor is essential for a positive and empowering childbirth experience. Providing continuous support, respectful care, effective pain management, clear communication, physical comfort, and psychological support can significantly enhance the overall experience for both the mother and the baby.

3. The second stage of labor

The second stage of labor begins when the cervix is fully dilated to 10 centimeters and ends with the birth of the baby. This stage is crucial as it involves the actual delivery of the baby through the birth canal [35].

3.1 Importance of the second stage of labor

1. Transition to birth: This stage marks the transition from labor to the birth of the baby. It is characterized by strong and regular contractions that help push the baby down the birth canal [36].

2. Maternal and neonatal outcomes: Proper management of this stage is vital for minimizing maternal and neonatal morbidity and mortality. A prolonged second stage can increase the risk of complications such as fetal distress and maternal exhaustion [37].

3. Physiological changes: The mother experiences significant physiological changes, including increased pressure on the rectum and the urge to push. These changes are essential for the successful delivery of the baby [38].

3.2 Care during the second stage of labor

1. Monitoring: Continuous monitoring of the fetal heart rate and maternal vital signs is crucial to ensuring the well-being of both mother and baby. This helps in early detection of any signs of distress [39].

2. Support and guidance: Providing emotional and physical support to the mother is essential. Encouraging words, helping with breathing techniques, and offering comfort measures such as changing positions can make a significant difference [40].

3. Pushing techniques: Guiding the mother with effective pushing techniques can help shorten the duration of the second stage and reduce the risk of complications. It is important to follow the mother's cues and allow her to push when she feels the urge [41].

4. Pain management: Pain relief options, such as epidurals or other analgesics, should be discussed and provided as per the mother's preference and medical advice [17].

5. Preventing perineal trauma: Measures to prevent perineal trauma, such as controlled pushing and the use of warm compresses, can help reduce the risk of tears and the need for episiotomy [42].

3.3 Complications in the second stage of labor

1. Prolonged labor: This occurs when the second stage of labor lasts longer than expected. Prolonged labor can increase the risk of maternal and fetal complications, including infection, postpartum hemorrhage, and the need for assisted delivery or cesarean section [43].

2. Fetal distress: This is a condition where the fetus does not receive adequate oxygen during labor, leading to abnormal heart rate patterns. Fetal distress can necessitate immediate interventions such as an emergency cesarean section [44].

3. Shoulder dystocia: This is a rare but serious complication where the baby's shoulder gets stuck behind the mother's pelvic bone after the head has been delivered. It requires prompt and skilled management to prevent injury to both the mother and baby [45].

4. Perineal trauma: Tears or lacerations to the perineum (the area between the vagina and the anus) are common during the second stage of labor. Severe tears can lead to significant pain, bleeding, and long-term complications such as incontinence [42].

5. Uterine rupture: Although rare, uterine rupture is a life-threatening complication where the uterine wall tears during labor. It is more common in women with a previous cesarean section or uterine surgery [46].

6. Maternal exhaustion: Prolonged pushing and labor can lead to significant physical and emotional exhaustion for the mother, impacting her ability to effectively participate in the delivery process [47].

In summary, the second stage of labor is a critical phase that requires careful management and support to ensure a safe and positive birth experience for both mother and baby. Midwifery support is crucial during the second stage of labor, as it can significantly impact the mother's experience and the outcome of the birth. Midwives provide both physical and emotional support, helping to ensure a safe and positive birthing experience [18].

DOI: http://dx.doi.org/10.5772/intechopen.1007173

4. The third stage of labor

The third stage of labor begins immediately after the birth of the baby and ends with the delivery of the placenta. This stage is crucial for ensuring the health and safety of both the mother and the newborn [1].

4.1 Importance of the third stage of labor

1. Placental separation and delivery: The primary event in this stage is the separation and expulsion of the placenta from the uterine wall. Proper management is essential to prevent complications such as retained placenta and excessive bleeding [48].

2. Prevention of postpartum hemorrhage: This stage is critical for preventing postpartum hemorrhage (PPH), which is a leading cause of maternal morbidity and mortality worldwide. Effective management can significantly reduce the risk of severe blood loss [49].

3. Uterine contraction: After the placenta is delivered, the uterus must contract to close off blood vessels and prevent hemorrhage. Ensuring strong uterine contractions is vital for minimizing blood loss [48].

4.2 Care during the third stage of labor

1. Active management: Active management of the third stage of labor (AMTSL) involves administering a uterotonic drug (usually oxytocin) immediately after the birth of the baby to stimulate uterine contractions and reduce the risk of PPH. This approach has been shown to decrease the incidence of severe hemorrhage and the need for blood transfusions [50].

   The important causes of postpartum bleeding can be summarized as four (T) [1]:

   - Tonicity (uterine atony after childbirth due to various causes such as long induction of labor, maternal obesity, and multiparity)
   - Trauma (caused by rupture of the uterus and genital tract)
   - Tissue (remaining placenta inside the uterus)
   - Thrombophilia (caused by disorders of blood coagulation factors)

2. Monitoring and assessment: Continuous monitoring of the mother's vital signs and blood loss is essential. Healthcare providers should assess the placenta to ensure it is complete and check for any signs of retained placental fragments [51].

3. Cord clamping: Delayed cord clamping (waiting 1–3 minutes after birth) is recommended to improve neonatal outcomes, including increased iron stores and reduced risk of anemia in the infant [1].

4. Perineal care: If an episiotomy was performed or if there were any perineal tears, they should be repaired promptly to prevent infection and promote healing [52].

5. Emotional support: Providing emotional support and reassurance to the mother during this stage is important. The birth of the baby can be overwhelming, and ensuring the mother feels supported can enhance her overall birth experience [53].

In summary, the third stage of labor is a critical period that requires careful management to ensure the health and safety of both the mother and the newborn. Active management, continuous monitoring, and providing emotional support are key components of care during this stage.

5. Four stages of labor

The fourth stage of labor, also known as the recovery stage, begins immediately after the delivery of the placenta and lasts for about two hours. This stage is crucial for monitoring the mother and ensuring that both she and the newborn are stable and healthy.

5.1 Importance of the fourth stage of labor

1. Monitoring for complications: This stage is critical for identifying and managing any immediate postpartum complications, such as postpartum hemorrhage, uterine atony, or retained placental fragments [54].

2. Uterine contraction: Ensuring that the uterus continues to contract is essential to prevent excessive bleeding. Uterine contractions help compress blood vessels and reduce the risk of hemorrhage [48].

3. Maternal and neonatal bonding: The fourth stage provides an opportunity for skin-to-skin contact between the mother and the newborn, which promotes bonding, stabilizes the baby's temperature, and encourages breastfeeding [55].

4. Assessment of vital signs: Continuous monitoring of the mother's vital signs, including blood pressure, pulse, and temperature, is important to detect any signs of distress or complications [56].

5.2 Care during the fourth stage of labor

1. Monitoring and assessment: Healthcare providers should closely monitor the mother's vital signs and uterine contractions. They should also assess the amount of vaginal bleeding and ensure that the uterus is firm and contracted.

2. Pain management: Providing appropriate pain relief is important to ensure the mother's comfort. This may include medications or nonpharmacological methods such as ice packs or warm compresses.

3. Emotional support: Offering emotional support and reassurance to the mother is crucial during this stage. The birth experience can be overwhelming, and providing a calm and supportive environment can help the mother feel more at ease [56].

4. Breastfeeding support: Encouraging and assisting the mother with breastfeeding during the fourth stage can help establish successful breastfeeding and promote the release of oxytocin, which aids in uterine contraction [57].

5. Perineal care: If the mother experiences any perineal tears or had an episiotomy, proper care and assessment of the perineal area are necessary to prevent infection and promote healing [58].

In summary, the fourth stage of labor is a critical period that requires careful monitoring and support to ensure the health and well-being of both the mother and the newborn. Effective management during this stage can help prevent complications and promote a positive postpartum experience.

6. Conclusion

The process of labor is divided into four distinct stages, each with its significance and required care to ensure the health and safety of both the mother and the newborn.

- First stage of labor: This stage involves the onset of labor and the dilation of the cervix. Proper monitoring and support during this stage are crucial for managing pain and ensuring the progress of labor.

- Second stage of labor: This stage begins with full cervical dilation and ends with the birth of the baby. Effective pushing techniques, continuous monitoring, and emotional support are essential to facilitate a safe delivery and minimize complications.

- Third stage of labor: This stage involves the delivery of the placenta. Active management, including the administration of uterotonic drugs, is important to prevent postpartum hemorrhage and ensure the complete expulsion of the placenta.

- Fourth stage of labor: Also known as the recovery stage, this period focuses on monitoring the mother and newborn for any immediate postpartum complications. Providing emotional support, pain management, and assistance with breastfeeding are key components of care during this stage.

Each stage of labor requires specific care and attention to ensure a positive and safe birthing experience. Continuous monitoring, effective pain management, and emotional support are critical throughout the entire process. By understanding and addressing the unique needs of each stage, healthcare providers can help mothers navigate labor with confidence and achieve the best possible outcomes for themselves and their babies.

Acknowledgements

I am very grateful to my dear husband (Rasoul Gurbanzadeh) and my children (Aysu and Araz) who accompanied me on this great and arduous journey of science. The author acknowledges the use of Grammarly AI tool for language polishing of the manuscript.

Conflict of interest

The author declares no conflict of interest.

Author details

Fatemeh Ahadi Yulghunlu
Faculty of Nursing and Midwifery, Department of Midwifery, Tabriz University of Medical Sciences, Tabriz, Iran

*Address all correspondence to: fatemehahadi8@gmail.com

References

[1] Gary Cunningham F, Leveno KJ, Dashe JS, Hoffman BL, Spong CY, Casey BM. Williams Obstetrics. Dallas, Texas: Mc Graw Hill Education; 2022. p. 26e

[2] Jayasundara D, Jayawardane IA, Weliange SDS, Jayasingha T, Madugalle T. Impact of continuous labor companion- who is the best: A systematic review and meta-analysis of randomized controlled trials. PLoS One. 2024;**19**(7):e0298852. DOI: 10.1371/journal.pone.0298852. Epub 2024/07/23

[3] Organization WHO. WHO Labour Care Guide User's Manual. Geneva, Switzerland: WHO; 2020

[4] Smith PA, Kilgour C, Rice D, Callaway LK, Martin EK. Implementation barriers and enablers of midwifery group practice for vulnerable women: A qualitative study in a tertiary urban Australian health service. BMC Health Services Research. 2022;**22**(1):1265

[5] NICE Evidence Reviews Collection. Evidence Reviews for Use of Oxytocin in the First or Second Stage of Labour: Intrapartum Care: Evidence Review F. London: National Institute for Health and Care Excellence (NICE) Copyright © NICE 2023; 2023

[6] Clinic M. Stages of labor and birth: Baby, it's time! Retrieved from Mayo Clinic. Rochester, Minnesota, USA: Mayo Clinic; 2024

[7] Hanley GE, Munro S, Greyson D, Gross MM, Hundley V, Spiby H, et al. Diagnosing onset of labor: A systematic review of definitions in the research literature. BMC Pregnancy and Childbirth. 2016;**16**:71. DOI: 10.1186/s12884-016-0857-4. Epub 2016/04/04

[8] What Are the Stages of Labor? [Internet]. 2024. Available from: https://www.nichd.nih.gov/health/topics/labor-delivery/topicinfo/stages

[9] Issac A, Nayak SG, Priyadarshini T, Balakrishnan D, Halemani K, Mishra P, et al. Effectiveness of breathing exercise on the duration of labour: A systematic review and meta-analysis. Journal of global health. 10 Mar 2023;**13**

[10] He X, Zeng X, Troendle J, Ahlberg M, Tilden EL, Souza JP, et al. New insights on labor progression: A systematic review. American Journal of Obstetrics and Gynecology. 2023;**228**(5):S1063-S1S94

[11] UpToDate. Labor and Delivery: Management of the Normal First Stage. 2024

[12] Feng Y, Zhu F, Zhang J, Zeng Z, Li Q. Efficacy of different strategies for reducing labor pain: A Bayesian analysis. Medicine. 2024;**103**(20):e37594. DOI: 10.1097/md.0000000000037594. Epub 2024/05/17

[13] Barut S, Sabancı Baransel E, Çelik OT, Uçar T. The trends and hotspots of research on non-pharmacological interventions for labor pain management: A bibliometric analysis. Journal of Psychosomatic Obstetrics and Gynaecology. 2024;**45**(1):2322614. DOI: 10.1080/0167482x.2024.2322614. Epub 2024/03/06

[14] Fadlalmola H, Abdelmalik MA, Masaad HKH, Abdalla AM, Mohammaed MO, Abbakr I, et al. Efficacy of warm compresses in preserving perineal integrity and decreasing pain during normal labor: A systematic review and meta-analysis. African Journal of Reproductive Health.

2023;**27**(4):96-123. DOI: 10.29063/ajrh2023/v27i4.11. Epub 2023/08/16

[15] Geltore TE, Alemu G, Taye A, Sileshi E, Bekele M, Foto LL. Determinants and willingness to practice obstetric analgesia among women attending antenatal clinic at Dr. Bogalech Gebre memorial general hospital Central Ethiopia: A cross-sectional study. BMC Pregnancy and Childbirth. 2024;**24**(1):470. DOI: 10.1186/s12884-024-06674-x. Epub 2024/07/11

[16] Zuarez-Easton S, Erez O, Zafran N, Carmeli J, Garmi G, Salim R. Pharmacologic and nonpharmacologic options for pain relief during labor: An expert review. American Journal of Obstetrics and Gynecology. 2023;**228**(5s):S1246-S1s59. DOI: 10.1016/j.ajog.2023.03.003. Epub 2023/04/03

[17] Tascón Padrón L, Emrich NLA, Strizek B, Schleußner E, Dreiling J, Komann M, et al. Quality of analgesic care in labor: A cross-sectional study of the first national register-based benchmarking system. International Journal of Gynaecology and Obstetrics: The Official Organ of the International Federation of Gynaecology and Obstetrics. 2024;**166**(3):1077-1085. DOI: 10.1002/ijgo.15489. Epub 2024/03/26

[18] Bradford BF, Wilson AN, Portela A, McConville F, Fernandez Turienzo C, Homer CS. Midwifery continuity of care: A scoping review of where, how, by whom and for whom? PLOS Global Public Health. 2022;**2**(10):e0000935

[19] Einion A. Hypnosis and hypnobirthing for labour – A critical selective narrative review. The Practising Midwife. 2016;**19**(11):25-27. Epub 2016/12/01

[20] Granger S. Hypnotherapy for childbirth. The Practising Midwife. 2012;**15**(8):S13-S14. Epub 2012/10/23

[21] Greenberg JT, Cross SN, Raab CA, Pettker CM, Illuzzi JL. Adherence to definitions of labor arrest influence on primary cesarean delivery rate. American Journal of Perinatology. 2024;**41**(5):618-627. DOI: 10.1055/a-1745-1570. Epub 2022/01/20

[22] Hamilton EF, Zhoroev T, Warrick PA, Tarca AL, Garite TJ, Caughey AB, et al. New labor curves of dilation and station to improve the accuracy of predicting labor progress. American Journal of Obstetrics and Gynecology. 2024;**231**(1):1-18. DOI: 10.1016/j.ajog.2024.02.289. Epub 2024/03/01

[23] Alhafez L, Berghella V. Evidence-based labor management: First stage of labor (part 3). American Journal of Obstetrics & Gynecology MFM. 2020;**2**(4):100185. DOI: 10.1016/j.ajogmf.2020.100185. Epub 2020/12/22

[24] Swer M Gl. The Continuous Textbook of Women's Medicine Series – Obstetrics Module. In: Chandraharan DE, editor. Labor and delivery. Springer Nature; 2021

[25] Gomes F, Ramalho C, Machado AP, Calado E, Cardoso F, Montenegro N. Transvaginal ultrasound assessment of the cervix and digital examination before labor induction. Acta Medica Portuguesa. 2006;**19**(2):109-114. Epub 2006/12/26

[26] Romero R. A profile of Emanuel a. Friedman, MD, DMedSci. American Journal of Obstetrics & Gynecology. 2016;**215**(4):413-414

[27] Ramadan MK, Fasih R, Itani S, Salem Wehbe GR, Badr DA. Characteristics of fetal and maternal heart rate tracings during labor: A prospective

observational study. Journal of Neonatal-Perinatal Medicine. 2019;**12**(4):405-410. DOI: 10.3233/npm-180044. Epub 2019/10/15

[28] Housseine N, Punt MC, Browne JL, van 't Hooft J, Maaløe N, Meguid T, et al. Delphi consensus statement on intrapartum fetal monitoring in low-resource settings. International Journal of Gynaecology and Obstetrics: The Official Organ of the International Federation of Gynaecology and Obstetrics. 2019;**146**(1):8-16. DOI: 10.1002/ijgo.12724. Epub 2018/12/26

[29] Schulten PS, Suppelna JP, Dagres T, Noè G, Anapolski M, Reinhard J, et al. Comparison of international guidelines for the application of Cardiotocography. Zeitschrift fur Geburtshilfe und Neonatologie. 2018;**222**(2):66-71. DOI: 10.1055/s-0043-122945. Epub 2018/02/24

[30] Meeting Women's Emotional, Psychological and Clinical Needs During Childbirth. 2020. Available from: https://www.who.int/news/item/20-08-2020-meeting-women-s-emotional-psychological-and-clinical-needs-during-childbirth

[31] Al-Mutawtah M, Campbell E, Kubis H-P, Erjavec M. Women's experiences of social support during pregnancy: A qualitative systematic review. BMC Pregnancy and Childbirth. 2023;**23**(1):782

[32] Combellick JL, Telfer ML, Ibrahim BB, Novick G, Morelli EM, James-Conterelli S, et al. Midwifery care during labor and birth in the United States. American Journal of Obstetrics and Gynecology. 2023;**228**(5):S983-SS93

[33] Lynam LE, Miller MA. Mothers' and nurses' perceptions of the needs of women experiencing preterm labor. Journal of Obstetric, Gynecologic, and Neonatal Nursing: JOGNN. 1992;**21**(2):126-136. DOI: 10.1111/j.1552-6909.1992.tb01731.x. Epub 1992/03/01

[34] Cooper M, Briley A, Feeley C, Dillon MF, McNeill ML, Medway MP, et al. Changin'it up: Shining the light on what it means to be informed in maternity care. Women and Birth. 2023;**36**:S44

[35] Häggsgård C, Edqvist M, Teleman P, Tern H, Rubertsson C. Impact of collegial midwifery assistance during second stage of labour on women's experience: A follow-up from the Swedish Oneplus randomised controlled trial. BMJ Open. 2024;**14**(7):e077458. DOI: 10.1136/bmjopen-2023-077458. Epub 2024/07/28

[36] Häggsgård C, Rubertsson C, Teleman P, Edqvist M. Informed consent to midwifery practices and interventions during the second stage of labor-an observational study within the Oneplus trial. PLoS One. 2024;**19**(6):e0304418. DOI: 10.1371/journal.pone.0304418. Epub 2024/06/12

[37] Niemczyk NA, Ren D, Stapleton SR. Associations between prolonged second stage of labor and maternal and neonatal outcomes in freestanding birth centers: A retrospective analysis. BMC Pregnancy and Childbirth. 2022;**22**(1):99. DOI: 10.1186/s12884-022-04421-8. Epub 2022/02/06

[38] Cohen WR, Friedman EA. The second stage of labor. American Journal of Obstetrics and Gynecology. 2024;**230**(3s):S865-Ss75. DOI: 10.1016/j.ajog.2022.06.014. Epub 2024/03/11

[39] Pizzagalli F. Normal childbirth: Physiologic labor support and medical procedures. Guidelines of the French National Authority for health (HAS) with the collaboration of the French

College of Gynaecologists and Obstetricians (CNGOF) and the French College of Midwives (CNSF) – Maternal postures during the second stage of labour, delivery techniques and perineal protection. Gynecologie, Obstetrique, Fertilite & Senologie. 2020;**48**(12):931-943. DOI: 10.1016/j.gofs.2020.09.018. Epub 2020/10/05

[40] Musie MR, Peu MD, Bhana-Pema V. Culturally appropriate care to support maternal positions during the second stage of labour: Midwives' perspectives in South Africa. African Journal of Primary Health Care & Family Medicine. 2022;**14**(1):e1-e9. DOI: 10.4102/phcfm.v14i1.3292. Epub 2022/05/10

[41] Cahill AG, Macones GA. Optimizing the length of the second stage and management of pushing. American Journal of Obstetrics and Gynecology. 2024;**230**(3s):S876-S8s8. DOI: 10.1016/j.ajog.2022.07.017. Epub 2024/03/11

[42] Saucedo AM, Tuuli MG, Gregory WT, Richter HE, Lowder JL, Woolfolk C, et al. First and second stage risk factors associated with perineal lacerations. Maternal and Child Health Journal. 2024;**28**(7):1228-1233. DOI: 10.1007/s10995-024-03919-1. Epub 2024/03/05

[43] Knigin D, Ezra Y, Ben-David A, Elami-Suzin M. The continuum of a prolonged labor and a second stage cesarean delivery. The Journal of Maternal-Fetal & Neonatal Medicine : The Official Journal of the European Association of Perinatal Medicine, the Federation of Asia and Oceania Perinatal Societies, the International Society of Perinatal Obstet. 2022;**35**(25):6425-6429. DOI: 10.1080/14767058.2021.1914577. Epub 2021/05/26

[44] Triebwasser JE, Colvin R, Macones GA, Cahill AG. Nonreassuring fetal status in the second stage of labor: Fetal monitoring features and association with neonatal outcomes. American Journal of Perinatology. 2016;**33**(7):665-670. DOI: 10.1055/s-0036-1571316. Epub 2016/02/11

[45] Marques JB, Reynolds A. Shoulder dystocia: An obstetrical emergency. Acta Medica Portuguesa. 2011;**24**(4):613-620. Epub 2012/04/24

[46] Deshmukh U, Denoble AE, Son M. Trial of labor after cesarean, vaginal birth after cesarean, and the risk of uterine rupture: An expert review. American Journal of Obstetrics and Gynecology. 2024;**230**(3s):S783-s803. DOI: 10.1016/j.ajog.2022.10.030. Epub 2024/03/11

[47] Ebrahimzadeh S, Golmakani N, Kabirian M, Shakeri MT. Study of correlation between maternal fatigue and uterine contraction pattern in the active phase of labour. Journal of Clinical Nursing. 2012;**21**(11-12):1563-1569. DOI: 10.1111/j.1365-2702.2012.04084.x. Epub 2012/04/24

[48] Abebe Gelaw K, Atalay YA, Azeze GA, Yitayew AM, Gebeyehu NA. Knowledge and factors associated with active management of the third stage of labor in sub-Saharan Africa: A systematic review and meta-analysis. International Journal of Gynaecology and Obstetrics: The Official Organ of the International Federation of Gynaecology and Obstetrics. 2024;**166**(3):943-953. DOI: 10.1002/ijgo.15560. Epub 2024/05/03

[49] Papadopoulou A, Tournas G, Georgiopoulos G, Antsaklis P, Daskalakis G, Coomarasamy A, et al. Preventing postpartum hemorrhage: A network meta-analysis on routes of administration of uterotonics. European Journal of Obstetrics, Gynecology, and

Reproductive Biology. 2024;**295**:172-180. DOI: 10.1016/j.ejogrb.2024.02.021. Epub 2024/02/18

[50] Mihretie GN, Ayele AD, Liyeh TM, Beyene FY, Kassa BG, Arega DT, et al. Active management of the third stage of labour in Ethiopia: A systematic review and meta-analysis. PLoS One. 2023;**18**(4):e0281343. DOI: 10.1371/journal.pone.0281343. Epub 2023/04/20

[51] Cohain JS. Novel third stage protocol https://www.youtube.com/watch?v=AAJPW4p6rzU reduces postpartum hemorrhage at vaginal birth. European Journal of Obstetrics, Gynecology, and Reproductive Biology. 2022;**278**:29-32. DOI: 10.1016/j.ejogrb.2022.08.016. Epub 2022/09/17

[52] NICE Evidence Reviews Collection. Evidence Reviews for Interventions to Reduce Perineal Trauma: Intrapartum Care: Evidence Review I. London: National Institute for Health and Care Excellence (NICE) Copyright © NICE 2023; 2023

[53] Rex J, Fifer N, Johnson-Webb KD, Menich M, Horn A, Salamone C, et al. "She's a family member": How community health workers impact perinatal Mothers' stress through social-emotional support and connections to programs and resources. Health Equity. 2024;**8**(1):469-479. DOI: 10.1089/heq.2024.0038. Epub 2024/07/16

[54] Kogner L, Lundborg L, Liu X, Ladfors LV, Ahlberg M, Stephansson O, et al. Duration of the active first stage of labour and severe perineal lacerations and maternal postpartum complications: A population-based cohort study. BJOG: An International Journal of Obstetrics and Gynaecology. 2024;**131**(6):832-842. DOI: 10.1111/1471-0528.17692. Epub 2023/10/16

[55] Shinohara S, Shinohara R, Kojima R, Otawa S, Kushima M, Miyake K, et al. Neonatal transfer and duration of hospitalization of newborns as potential risk factors for impaired mother-infant bonding: The Japan environment and Children's study. Journal of Affective Disorders. 2024;**360**:314-321. DOI: 10.1016/j.jad.2024.06.001. Epub 2024/06/06

[56] Adams YJ, Miller ML, Agbenyo JS, Ehla EE, Clinton GA. Postpartum care needs assessment: women's understanding of postpartum care, practices, barriers, and educational needs. BMC Pregnancy and Childbirth. 2023;**23**(1):502

[57] Shipton EV, Callaway L, Foxcroft K, Lee N, de Jersey SJ. Midwife-led continuity of antenatal care and breastfeeding duration beyond postpartum hospital discharge: A systematic review. Journal of Human Lactation. 2023;**39**(3):427-440

[58] Girsang BM, Elfira E. Development of a web-based "perineal care protocol" educational model as assistance for postpartum perineal wound care at home. Family Medicine & Primary Care Review. 2023;**25**(2):160-164

Chapter 7

Prevention and Management of Postpartum Hemorrhage

Rebecca Bradley and Alexander Juusela

Abstract

Postpartum hemorrhage remains a prevalent and potentially life-threatening obstetric emergency, historically representing a leading cause of maternal mortality among women of reproductive age. Although advancements in clinical and medical technology have contributed to a global reduction in maternal mortality rates, sustaining and further improving these outcomes necessitates proactive, standardized, and evidence-based approaches to obstetric care. Effective prevention and management of postpartum hemorrhage require systematic efforts to control modifiable risk factors through the implementation of standardized, evidence-based care protocols; structured education; simulation-based training; provider awareness; proactive clinical management; and care bundles. These strategies are critical to optimizing maternal outcomes, reducing morbidity, and preventing obstetric hemorrhage-related mortality. This chapter provides a comprehensive review of the prevention and management of postpartum hemorrhage from both individual patient and population health perspectives. It addresses fundamental concepts, risk factors, key determinants, and evidence-based solutions. This chapter is intended for educational purposes and is not designed to serve as a guide for the clinical management of the conditions described; thus, discussions of management are intentionally brief. The information provided is intended for general knowledge and should not be used to diagnose or treat a medical condition without consultation from a qualified healthcare provider. This chapter is not a substitute for professional medical advice, diagnosis, or treatment.

Keywords: maternal mortality, maternal death, obstetrical labor, complications, obstetric emergency, postpartum hemorrhage, pregnancy, labor, quality improvement, public health, maternal health, hemorrhage, postpartum hemorrhage risk factors, postpartum hemorrhage-related mortality, prenatal anemia, bleeding, essential medicines, surgery, trauma, c-section, cesarean section, childbirth

1. Introduction

The *maternal mortality ratio*, defined as "the number of maternal deaths per 100,000 live births," has been a subject of much scrutiny throughout the world, but especially, most recently, in the United States. Despite spending more money per capita on health care, the United States consistently has a higher rate of maternal mortality than other high-income and developed countries [1]. According to the CDC, the maternal mortality ratio in the United States has increased between 2018 and 2022, from 17.3 to 22.3 maternal deaths per 100,000 live births [2]. The most drastic increase was between 2020 and 2021, likely directly and indirectly due to the coronavirus pandemic. Most maternal deaths are generally considered preventable, and so it is prudent to evaluate the most common causes of maternal mortality as well as ways to mitigate them in order to make a noticeable change [1].

One of the most common etiologies leading to severe maternal morbidity and mortality is postpartum hemorrhage. *Postpartum hemorrhage (PPH)*, defined as "cumulative blood loss of greater than or equal to 1,000 mL or blood loss accompanied by signs or symptoms of hypovolemia within 24 hours after the birth process," accounts for about 10% of maternal deaths in the United States [3]. It is also one of the leading causes of severe maternal morbidity in the United States and is the leading cause of maternal mortality worldwide [4]. While there is a lack of data on the rates of PPH stratified by state in the United States, extrapolating from data on maternal mortality by state, there is likely a higher postpartum hemorrhage rate in the states with higher poverty rates and lower maternal resources.

As PPH contributes to the increased maternal mortality rate and severe morbidity in pregnancy in the United States, a focus on prevention, early recognition, and swift management may help to decrease the incidence of maternal death or permanent sequelae.

2. Risk factors and etiology of postpartum hemorrhage

Risk factors for postpartum hemorrhage and the requirement for blood transfusion are well defined in the literature. These can be stratified into pregnancy-related etiologies such as placental abruption, abnormal placentation, intrauterine fetal demise, and severe preeclampsia/HELLP syndrome, as well as inherent factors such as age >34 years and being Black, Hispanic, and Asian/Pacific Islander [5].

Postpartum hemorrhage can be grouped into two categories based on how far out from delivery a woman is. *Primary postpartum hemorrhage* occurs within 24 h of birth and accounts for the majority of PPH cases [6]. *Secondary postpartum hemorrhage* occurs greater than 24 h after delivery and up to 12 weeks postpartum [6]. Risk factors for postpartum hemorrhage can also be stratified by primary and secondary causes. Risk factors/etiology for primary postpartum hemorrhage include abnormalities of uterine contraction, genital tract trauma, retained placental tissue, and abnormalities of coagulation. Secondary causes of postpartum hemorrhage include subinvolution of the placental site, retained products of conception, infection, and inherited coagulation defects [4, 6].

A helpful mnemonic for the causes of primary postpartum hemorrhage that has been widely used is the *"Four T's" of postpartum hemorrhage*: *Tone* (atonic uterus), *Trauma* (lacerations, hematomas, uterine inversion or rupture), *Tissue* (retained placenta or abnormal placentation), and *Thrombin* (coagulopathies) (**Figure 1**) [7].

These etiologies can be further broken down by the risk factor that causes them. It is important to identify these risk factors and plan for the potential complication of excessive bleeding in order to mitigate the morbidity associated with hemorrhage.

2.1 Abnormalities of uterine contraction (tone)

Uterine atony, or failure of the uterus to contract after delivery, is by far the most common cause of primary postpartum hemorrhage, accounting for approximately

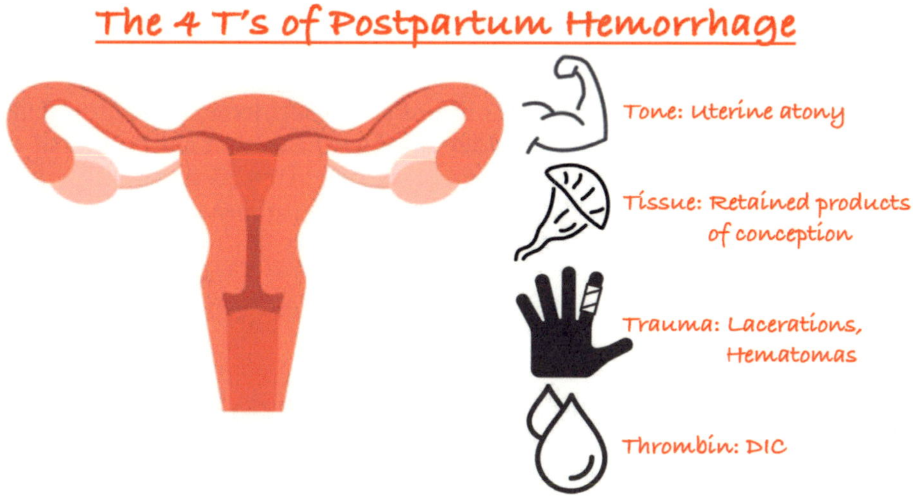

Figure 1.
The 4T's of postpartum hemorrhage.

80% of cases [8]. There are multiple factors that can contribute to abnormal uterine contraction following delivery. Anything that over distends the uterus, such as multiple gestations, distortion of the uterus (multiple fibroids, uterine anomalies), macrosomia, or polyhydramnios, has the potential to affect contractility. Other factors that can contribute to inhibition of normal contraction of the uterus are prolonged oxytocin administration, increased parity, chorioamnionitis, and being given general anesthesia during cesarean section [7].

Adequate uterine tone requires the muscle cells of the myometrium to contract properly in response to oxytocin stimulation following delivery. The muscle cell of the myometrium stays at resting potential due to the maintenance of intracellular and extracellular K+ and Na+ ions [9]. Myometrial contraction is caused by an action potential in the cell that results in an influx of Na+ intracellularly, which is referred to as "electromagnetic coupling" [9]. During pregnancy, the spiral arteries that provide blood flow to the placenta lose their smooth muscle and therefore require the contraction of the myometrium to prevent blood loss after delivery [9]. If there are factors during labor and delivery that negatively influence the contractility of the myometrium, PPH hemorrhage can occur. Medications that facilitate the contraction of the uterus are therefore used as first-line treatment for postpartum hemorrhage.

2.1.1 Uterine inversion

Uterine inversion is a rare and potentially life-threatening complication of vaginal delivery that occurs when there is complete or partial inversion of the uterine fundus into the endometrial cavity in the third stage of labor. It has an incidence of approximately 2.9 per 10,000 deliveries [10]. This can occur due to excessive cord traction while waiting for delivery of the placenta, a short umbilical cord, or abnormal placentation such as placenta accreta spectrum disorders [10]. In a large multicenter study, the rate of PPH secondary to uterine inversion was 37%, the rate of blood transfusion was 22.4%, and the requirement for surgical intervention was 6% [10]. Due to the high incidence of severe morbidity associated with uterine inversion, early recognition and management are essential. An inverted uterus can sometimes present as a bluish-gray mass protruding from the vagina after delivery [7]. However, in cases of incomplete inversion, it can be harder to identify. Therefore, when faced with excessive bleeding without an identifiable cause, practitioners should ensure to rule out uterine inversion. This highlights the role of having all births attended by skilled obstetricians or obstetric providers in order to reduce the risks of morbidity and mortality. In the event of this rare complication, access to medication such as uterine relaxants and the ability to undergo swift surgical intervention are crucial. In rural or low-resource hospitals, without access to these interventions, delays in care may result in severe maternal morbidity and mortality.

2.2 Genital tract trauma (trauma)

Any injury to the vaginal canal, cervix, uterus, or anal sphincters increases the risk of PPH. The risk for perineal, vaginal, and cervical lacerations is increased when episiotomy is performed, with precipitous deliveries, or with operative vaginal delivery [6]. These interventions should therefore not be routinely performed, and care should be taken to mitigate the risks of lacerations and trauma. If these interventions are performed, the vaginal vault, cervix, and perineum should be evaluated thoroughly following delivery, and if indicated, ensure prompt repair to minimize blood loss.

2.2.1 Uterine rupture

Uterine rupture is a rare complication of labor that generally occurs when a patient with a uterine scar from a previous cesarean section [7] or previous uterine surgery, such as a myomectomy, undergoes labor. The rate of uterine rupture with one prior low transverse cesarean delivery is approximately 0.5–0.9% [11]. Uterine rupture can be identified by abnormalities of the fetal heart rate, loss of fetal station, a sudden lack of contractions on the tocodynamometry, a change in maternal pain sensation, as well as vaginal bleeding [7]. Surgical repair of the defect is required to minimize blood loss and complications [7]. A high index of suspicion and prompt treatment of suspected uterine rupture will decrease the risks of severe maternal and neonatal morbidity and mortality from uterine rupture and hemorrhage. Rarely, uterine rupture occurs in unscarred uteruses, with an incidence of 0.2 per 10,000 births [12]. This can occur as a complication of distorted anatomy of the uterus, such as a bicornuate uterus, uterine septum, or fibroid uterus [12].

2.3 Tissue

2.3.1 Retained products of conception

Retained placenta is defined as failure of the placenta to separate and deliver within 30 min after birth and occurs in approximately 3% of vaginal deliveries [7]. The average time from delivery of the neonate to delivery of the placenta is 8–9 min, and the rate of hemorrhage increases with increasing time from delivery after 10 min [7]. If the placenta does not deliver after 30 min, injection of the umbilical cord with 20 mL of 0.9% saline and 20 units of oxytocin will sometimes reduce the need for manual removal of the placenta [7]. If this does not work, manual removal of the placenta can be attempted [7]. If there is no plane identifiable between the uterus and the placenta,

placenta accreta spectrum (PAS) should be suspected. Prompt identification of PAS can decrease the risk of severe morbidity and mortality in these cases [13].

2.3.2 Placenta accreta spectrum

Placenta accreta spectrum (PAS) disorders have been increasing in incidence, likely due to the increase in cesarean deliveries in the United States, with the overall incidence now approaching 0.17% of all pregnancies [13]. The most significant risk factor for PAS is placenta previa in a patient with a history of cesarean section or other uterine manipulation, such as myomectomy or uterine instrumentation, such as multiple D&Cs [13]. PAS will also be increased with a history of Asherman syndrome or endometrial ablation, multifetal gestation, and IVF pregnancies [13]. PAS is a spectrum of disorders of abnormal placentation and encompasses placenta accreta or Grade 1 PAS (areas of abnormal decidua between the villi and myometrium), placenta increta or Grade 2 PAS (irregular myometrium interface without involvement of outer myometrium), and placenta increta/percreta or Grade 3 PAS (irregular placenta-myometrium interface to the outer myometrium—3A, deep myometrial invasion—3D, or extrauterine extension—3E) [13].

Ideally, PAS would be diagnosed prior to delivery; however, diagnostic tools such as ultrasound often do not accurately predict or diagnose PAS, which can increase the risk of incidental PAS on delivery. This increases the risk of PPH and subsequent morbidity and mortality, especially in low-resource settings [13]. Patients with high-risk pregnancies, such as those with multiple cesarean deliveries or placenta previa, should ideally be sent for additional imaging and evaluation of the placenta multiple times in pregnancy [13]. However, in low socioeconomic settings, the logistics of this may be difficult, as patients often do not have reliable transportation, childcare, or other support necessary to get to these appointments. All of these factors may be contributing to the high incidence of undiagnosed PAS in up to 50% of cases [13]. In low-resource settings, especially, being prepared for PAS may decrease morbidity and mortality related to PPH. There are readiness and response checklists available from the Society of Maternal Fetal Medicine website that can be used to create policies surrounding undiagnosed PAS [13]. If PAS is suspected prior to delivery, transfer to a tertiary care center may improve outcomes at low-resource hospitals [13].

2.4 Thrombin

Disorders of coagulation are the last subset of risk factors that are associated with PPH, and, while rare, they are unlikely to respond to normal measures used to correct postpartum bleeding. Identifying these disorders prior to delivery is paramount for treatment purposes [7]. Disorders under this umbrella are inherited or autoimmune disorders of coagulation, such as Von Willebrand disease, idiopathic thrombocytopenic purpura, and thrombocytopenic purpura, as well as pregnancy-related disorders of coagulation such as HELLP syndrome, acute fatty liver of pregnancy, and amniotic fluid embolism. There are also infectious causes of disseminated intravascular coagulation (DIC), such as prolonged chorioamnionitis, prolonged retention of fetal demise, or placental abruption [7]. Increased suspicion for coagulation disorders should arise when the patient has been inspected for trauma, is not responding to the normal interventions for PPH, or is not forming clots appropriately [7]. Inherited or autoimmune disorders of coagulation can often be diagnosed prior to delivery with a good history and physical, including family history of bleeding disorders, or by evaluation of antenatal blood work for abnormalities such as severe thrombocytopenia [7].

3. Prevention of PPH

As PPH is one of the complications of pregnancy with one of the highest morbidity and mortality rates, focus on prevention should be at the forefront in efforts to reduce complications of pregnancy overall. Risk factors for PPH should be identified prior to delivery, and strategies to minimize the effects of PPH should be undertaken when appropriate. These strategies include correcting anemia prior to delivery, being aware of the mother's desires when it comes to blood transfusions, and eliminating routine episiotomy [7]. Routine inspection of the genital tract and repair of lacerations after operative vaginal delivery may also identify trauma that could potentially cause excessive bleeding if not identified quickly [7].

While it is impossible to prevent postpartum hemorrhage in all cases, active management of the 3rd stage of labor is one of the most widely used preventive strategies to reduce the incidence of PPH [7]. These interventions can be implemented at any hospital that has the capability of doing deliveries and has been shown to decrease the incidence of PPH significantly over expectant management [7].

Cord traction, as compared to expectant management for delivery of the placenta, can shorten the third stage of labor as well as decrease the risk of PPH by up to 68% [7]. This can be done by any delivering provider regardless of the setting or resources of the hospital and, as such, may decrease the disparity that can be seen in low-resource settings. Uterine massage is another intervention that has been shown to decrease postpartum bleeding. Although the data regarding uterine massage and its overall effect on PPH is conflicting, one study showed that uterine massage performed every 10 min after delivery of the placenta decreased the need for additional uterotonics by about 80% [14]. Uterine massage facilitates continued contraction of the uterus. It does not require any additional resources aside from a nurse or provider capable of doing so, and is therefore another low-cost intervention that should be performed with all deliveries.

Prophylactic administration of a tocolytic agent after delivery of the placenta has been shown to reduce the rate of postpartum hemorrhage by 40%. Oxytocin is by far the most widely used in the United States due to its effectiveness and fewer side effects than other uterotonic agents [7]. Oxytocin can be administered either before or after delivery of the placenta, as timing of administration has not been shown to be significant on its overall effectiveness [7]. Oxytocin can be administered by dilute intravenous infusion with a bolus dose of 10 units or by IM injection of 10 units. Oxytocin in some form is recommended for every delivery performed in the United States, regardless of the route of delivery [15].

4. Management of PPH

While identifying risk factors and utilizing risk stratification tools may decrease the incidence and severity of PPH, it is impossible to eliminate the incidence of postpartum hemorrhage entirely. Therefore, early recognition and management of excessive bleeding are important in decreasing the morbidity and mortality associated with PPH [7]. Postpartum care should include routine evaluation of uterine tone,

Medication	Dosage	Interval	Contraindications
Oxytocin	10–40 units per 500–1000 mL IV or 10 units IM	Continuous infusion. Once	Hypersensitivity
Methylergonivine	0.20 mg IM	Every 2–4 h	Hypersensitivity, hypertension, preeclampsia, cardiovascular disease
Prostaglandin F2α	0.25 mg IM	Every 15–90 min (maximum of 2 mg or eight doses)	Absolute: Asthma Relative: Active hepatic, pulmonary, or cardiac disease
Misoprostol	600–1000 mcg PO, sublingual, or rectal	Once	Hypersensitivity
Tranexamic acid	1 gram IV over 10 to 20 min	May repeat once in 30 min if bleeding continues.	Active intravascular clotting, active thromboembolic disease, subarachnoid hemorrhage

Table 1.
Medications for the prevention and management of postpartum hemorrhage.

vital signs, and vaginal bleeding in order to quickly identify patients that may need treatment in order to minimize the risk of severe hypovolemia [15]. When excessive bleeding is identified, the provider should quickly evaluate the vagina, cervix, and uterus to attempt to determine the etiology. Management of PPH starts with the least invasive (bimanual massage and medication interventions (**Table 1**)) to the most invasive (surgical intervention such as intrauterine balloon tamponade, B-Lynch sutures, or hysterectomy) [15].

4.1 Uterine atony

Uterine atony is the most common cause of postpartum hemorrhage, and any institution that provides maternal care should have policies and procedures in place in order to manage this delivery complication. Standard management of uterine atony starts with uterine massage, which entails manually compressing the uterine fundus by placing one hand in the vagina and the other hand externally against the anterior abdominal wall. The two hands compress the uterus and massage the anterior and posterior aspects of the uterus, which stimulates it to contract and improve uterine tone [6, 7].

4.1.1 Oxytocin

Oxytocin is the first-line uterotonic drug recommended for the treatment of PPH and should be administered at every delivery [7]. It can be administered intramuscularly or intravenously while bimanual/uterine massage is being performed [15, 16]. If oxytocin and bimanual massage do not adequately contract the uterus, other uterotonics should be considered.

4.1.2 Methylergonovine

Methylergonovine is an ergot alkaloid that causes smooth muscle contraction and, therefore, is given to contract the uterus in the event of PPH caused by uterine atony [7]. This is generally given as a second-line medication after oxytocin. It can be administered into the uterine muscle during cesarean section or intramuscularly after vaginal delivery in a dose of 0.2 mg [7]. Repeat doses can be administered at 2–4 h intervals, as necessary, to control bleeding [7]. Methergine is contraindicated in patients with hypertension and therefore cannot be used in patients with preexisting hypertension or hypertensive disorders of pregnancy, including preeclampsia [6, 7, 17].

4.1.3 Prostaglandin F2α

Prostaglandin F2α is a prostaglandin that increases contractility and vasoconstriction of the uterus and has been shown to control hemorrhage in up to 87% of PPH cases [7]. It is also used as a second-line medication after oxytocin and uterine massage to control postpartum bleeding. It can be repeated in 15-minute increments up to a total dose of 2 mg. While not an absolute contraindication, it is generally accepted that it should not be used in patients with asthma, as it can cause exacerbation [7]. It can also cause GI disturbance, such as diarrhea [6, 7].

4.1.4 Misoprostol

Misoprostol is another prostaglandin, used if the aforementioned medications do not control bleeding. It is generally given rectally in a dose of 1000 mcg [7]. It is considered third line after the previously mentioned medications, as it can take some time to absorb through the rectal mucosa and therefore does not act as fast as the IV/IM or intrauterine administrations. However, it can be given second-line if there are contraindications to either prostaglandin F2α or methergine [7, 13].

4.1.5 Tranexamic acid

Tranexamic acid is a synthetic, reversible, competitive inhibitor of the lysine receptor found on plasminogen. Once bound to plasmin, the active form of plasminogen, it assists in stabilizing the fibrin matrix. Tranexamic acid is administered 1 g intravenously over 10–20 min. It can be re-dosed once in 30 min if bleeding continues. Since the publication of the WOMAN trial (World Maternal Antifibrinolytic Trial), tranexamic acid, an antifibrinolytic drug, can provide a "complimentary effect" if co-administered with oxytocin and can help treat bleeding in the event of hemorrhage, providing up to 10 h of increased hemostasis after delivery [3]. It is recommended that TXA be administered as soon as possible after the diagnosis of PPH is made, and up to 3 h after delivery [15].

4.2 Hemorrhage bundles

It is recommended that a hemorrhage cart containing all of these medications be available for every delivery and be part of a safety bundle used for maternal safety developed by the National Partnership for Maternal Safety in 2015 [15]. The hemorrhage cart is part of the "readiness" component of the action plans outlined in this bundle [15]. The other three action domains are recognition and prevention, response, and reporting/systems learning [15]. FIGO recommends implementing postpartum hemorrhage bundles to improve and streamline care of PPH at any facility that does deliveries [15]. A 2024 systematic review analyzed the effectiveness of different care bundles for the prevention and treatment of postpartum hemorrhage and found heterogeneous results, with certain bundles demonstrating benefits, such as decreased hemorrhage rates; however, the optimal care bundle configuration was not identified [18].

4.3 Non-medication interventions

If postpartum hemorrhage cannot be controlled via medication interventions, consideration should be given to internal compression via intrauterine balloon tamponade or vacuum-induced hemorrhage-control devices, such as the Jada System [19]. These intermediary interventions can prevent the need for escalation to surgical interventions and have been shown to control bleeding in 87% and 94% of cases, respectively [19].

Once medication and tamponade techniques have been utilized and bleeding is still heavy, in hemodynamically stable patients, uterine artery embolization can be attempted. This is a fertility-sparing procedure and has success rates of approximately 85–95% [20]. This procedure involves embolization of the anterior trunk of the internal iliac arteries under fluoroscopic guidance by an interventional radiologist [20]. This is only an option at facilities with these resources, which may limit access for patients who live in rural or underserved areas. Vascular perfusion to the embolized vessels returns over time, and so future childbearing is usually preserved [20]. The caveat is that uterine artery embolization can only be attempted if the patient is stable and does not show signs of hypovolemic shock [20], which can limit its usefulness at this point in the management algorithm.

4.4 Surgical interventions

If conservative interventions fail to control bleeding, the next step in postpartum hemorrhage in the setting of uterine atony is surgical intervention. Uterine compression sutures are the first surgical procedure that can be tried and are a more conservative option that can be done prior to hysterectomy. Uterine compression sutures have the added benefit of preserving fertility [20]. There are multiple surgical options for uterine compression; however, the most commonly used compression suture is the B-Lynch suture [21]. A delayed-absorbable suture is anchored to the lower uterine segment, the uterus is folded onto itself, then the suture is passed over the fundus to create two "suspender"-like longitudinal bands that compress the uterus mechanically [21]. This can have a success rate as high as >75%, although studies are limited and the success rates vary [21, 22].

When uterine compression sutures fail, the next surgical step should be uterine artery ligation. The most commonly used technique is the O'Leary technique, where bilateral sutures are used to ligate the ascending branches of the uterine arteries [22]. This is sometimes done in conjunction with compression sutures in order to decrease the incidence of failed surgical management [22]. Alternative methods include Tsirulnikov's triple ligation [23] and the AbdRabbo's stepwise uterine devascularization [24].

Internal iliac (hypogastric) artery ligation was first described in 1898 [25] and has been demonstrated to be on average 69% effective [published range 39–100%] at controlling postpartum hemorrhage [26]. Hypogastric artery ligation requires exploration of the posterior peritoneal space and circumferential dissection of the anterior branch of the internal iliac artery, with ligation performed 2 cm below the iliac bifurcation, with care not to accidentally ligate the posterior branch, which supplies the gluteus muscles. This procedure must be performed bilaterally in order to achieve hemostasis.

If all of these interventions fail, the final step in the management of postpartum hemorrhage is the definitive management of hysterectomy [20]. The need for hysterectomy in the peripartum period is most commonly due to uterine atony and abnormal placentation and occurs in approximately 0.8 in 1000 deliveries [20]. In the event that all other interventions have failed and hysterectomy is deemed necessary, it should not be delayed, as continued bleeding could lead to DIC and death [20]. These hysterectomies can be technically very difficult due to the changes in anatomy during pregnancy, including large dilated vessels and increased vasculature to the uterus [20].

Uterine atony is the most common cause of postpartum hemorrhage; however, if this is not the etiology, quickly identifying and treating the underlying cause is paramount. In the event of uterine inversion, if the placenta remains attached to the endometrium, it should not be removed until the uterus is reduced to avoid additional bleeding [7]. If the placenta does remain attached, there should be consideration that this could be caused by abnormal placentation and managed accordingly [27]. Management of uterine inversion aims at replacing the uterus to its normal anatomic position as quickly as possible to minimize bleeding [7, 28]. Medications to relax the contraction of the uterus, such as magnesium sulfate or nitroglycerin, can facilitate replacement [7]. One method of uterine replacement, the Johnson method, involves grasping the uterine fundus and exerting force toward the posterior fornix and then up toward the umbilicus [7]. Once the uterus is replaced into anatomic position, uterotonics may be given to prevent recurrence [7, 27]. If the uterus is unable to be replaced manually, surgical intervention is necessary. There are two procedures used to replace the uterus surgically, the Huntington and Haultain procedures [27]. The Huntington procedure involves grasping the round ligaments on either side and gradually walking the uterus back into its anatomical position [27]. If the cervical ring is too tight, the Haultain procedure can be used to incise the cervical ring posteriorly in order to facilitate replacement [27]. If abnormal placentation is diagnosed, hysterectomy is the definitive management [7, 27].

If genital tract trauma is the cause of the bleeding, repair of the laceration or management of hematoma will minimize or stop the blood loss [7]. Small hematomas can be managed expectantly with pain medication, ice packs, and pressure [7]. If the hematoma is expanding, opening the area and ligating bleeding vessels may be necessary [7].

4.5 Coagulation defects

Ideally, coagulation defects are diagnosed antepartum, and multidisciplinary plans are made for delivery in order to mitigate the risk of bleeding. A good history and physical can identify patients who need extra testing for these disorders; however, not all coagulation defects are inherited or have noticeable symptoms prior to pregnancy [7, 29]. Additionally, some coagulation defects, such as DIC, are acquired after acute blood loss [29]. In the setting of postpartum hemorrhage that does not have an identifiable cause, or when bleeding is brisk and not clotting, coagulopathy should be considered [7]. Laboratory testing, including coagulation factors, early in a PPH can help direct appropriate management options. If disordered coagulation is the cause, treatment specific to that coagulopathy is warranted [7].

Fibrinogen may be used to assess the severity of postpartum hemorrhage and help diagnose a consumptive coagulopathy [28, 29]. Fibrinogen is typically doubled or more in pregnancy, which may delay diagnosis of coagulopathy, as traditionally low levels of fibrinogen under 200 mg/dL are generally not seen in pregnancy until extremely dangerous levels of consumption have occurred [28–30]. Outside of pregnancy, maintaining fibrinogen levels >100 mg/dL has been shown to maintain hemostasis; however, this number is likely too low in pregnancy, and a standard pregnancy level has not been established [28]. Disseminated intravascular coagulation (DIC) can be defined as "an acquired syndrome characterized by the intravascular activation of coagulation with a loss of localization arising from different causes. It can originate from and cause damage to the microvasculature, which if sufficiently severe, can produce organ dysfunction" [30]. Laboratory studies show thrombocytopenia, prolonged PT/PTT, low fibrinogen, and elevated D-Dimers [30]. Management of DIC should be focused on the underlying cause and is generally through a massive transfusion protocol [30], which will be discussed in the subsequent section.

5. Massive obstetric hemorrhage

Due to the normal physiologic changes in pregnancy, the expected signs and symptoms of hypovolemia in non-pregnant individuals may not be evident until there has been a large amount of blood loss in the pregnant patient [17]. In pregnancy, there is a large increase in plasma volume, as well as increased cardiac output, which can mask symptoms of anemia due to acute blood loss [17]. Pregnancy is also a state of physiologic hypercoagulability due to increased plasma concentrations of clotting factors, such as fibrinogen, and decreased anticoagulation factors, such as protein S (**Table 2**) [17]. These physiologic changes can lead to decreased recognition of consumptive coagulopathy and delay in management.

Physiologic changes in the coagulation system during pregnancy	Change in pregnancy
Procoagulants	
Factor II	No change
Factor V	No change
Factor VII	↑
Factor VIII	↑
Factor IX	No change
Factor X	↑
Fibrinogen	↑
Plasminogen Activation Inhibitor-1	↑
Plasminogen Activation Inhibitor-2	↑
Von Willebrand Factor (vWF)	↑
Anticoagulants	
Antithrombin	No change
Free Protein S	↓
Protein C	No change

Table 2.
Physiologic changes in the coagulation system during pregnancy.

While data that specifically analyzes massive hemorrhage in the obstetric setting is limited, data regarding massive hemorrhage and blood transfusion in the general surgical setting can be extrapolated for use in obstetrics [5, 17]. Massive transfusion is generally defined as the transfusion of 10 or more units of packed red blood cells in less than 24 h [17]. This type of mobilization can be extremely taxing on smaller hospitals with lower resources and may increase morbidity in low-income areas [5].

Abnormal placentation has the strongest association with the need for massive transfusion, with approximately 1.4% of patients with abnormal placentation requiring massive transfusion [5]. If abnormal placentation or another indication for peripartum hysterectomy is suspected prior to delivery, maternal morbidity and mortality may be decreased if the patient is delivered at a tertiary care center with more resources [5].

The first step in the management of massive obstetric hemorrhage is prompt recognition, two large-bore IVs, and early administration of IV fluids (**Figure 2**) [17]. Activation of a massive transfusion protocol (MTP) is generally done by the physician or delivering practitioner at the bedside, which triggers the blood bank to send blood products in a ratio of 1:1 RBCs to fresh frozen plasma (FFP), although the exact number of units and ratio remains subject to discussion, and there are very few formal recommendations [31]. One limitation to acquiring these blood products is that FFP takes some time to thaw, and in an emergency, this delay can increase complications. Some institutions have created protocols where varying numbers of FFP units are thawed automatically in the event of an emergency [31], and it should be a consideration at any hospital capable of providing pregnancy-related care.

6. Improving care in the setting of postpartum hemorrhage

Numerous studies have been conducted to identify effective strategies for improving the management of postpartum hemorrhage and reducing its associated morbidity and mortality, with the goal of standardizing care protocols. There should be processes in place when hemorrhage is recognized, and drills should be run often so that all members of the obstetrical team are aware and ready when a hemorrhage occurs [32]. Early identification and management of the specific etiology, as aforementioned, can prevent significant hemorrhage and its sequelae. Massive transfusion protocols have been shown to facilitate rapid treatment of hemorrhage as well as improve communication during a hemorrhagic emergency [5, 17, 32].

7. Systems-related factors that contribute to quality care in the setting of PPH

There are many potential quality issues that are highlighted when patients have postpartum hemorrhage. According to Jerome J. Federspiel et al., there are three "systems level factors" that can contribute to impaired quality of care in these cases [32].

7.1 Systems-related factor 1: Access to care

The first key factor is access to care [32]. The state of healthcare and lack of resources in many areas of the United States limit access to qualified doctors and midwives who are able to give the kind of quality care necessary to mitigate risk and

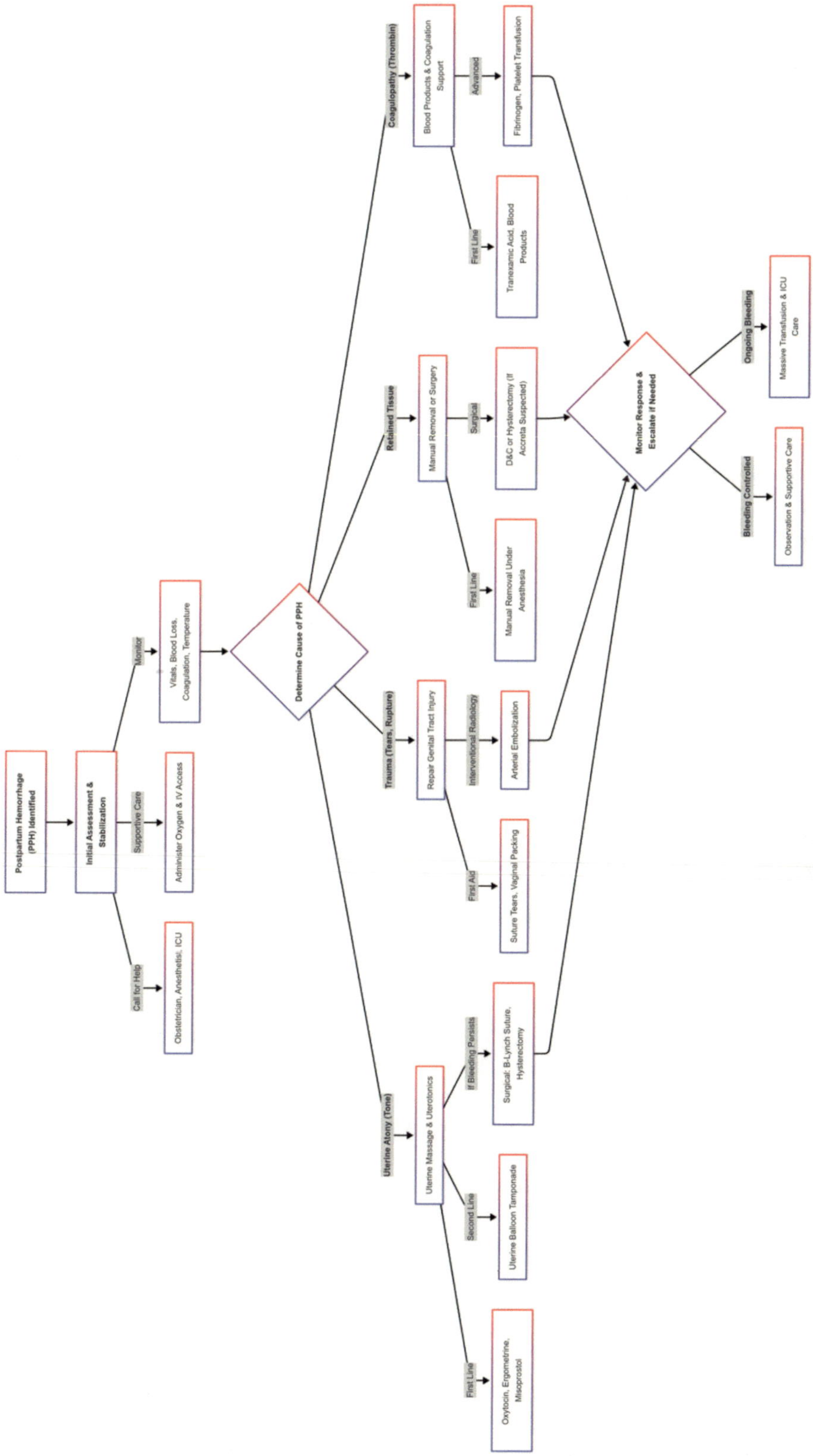

Figure 2.
Algorithm for the treatment and management of postpartum hemorrhage.

manage PPH swiftly. An estimated 2 million women in the United States live in a "*maternal care desert,*" defined as a location where access to reproductive care services, including maternity health care services, is absent or limited [31, 33, 34]. A true maternity desert has no hospital that is able to provide obstetric care, and a limited-access area has two or less than two hospitals with these services [31].

Maternity deserts arise due to multiple factors, including legislation that prohibits effective care and/or creates an environment in which Ob/Gyns feel compelled to leave or avoid practicing [33, 34]. As of 2021, approximately one-third of American women live in a county defined as a maternity care desert [33, 34], and this has, and likely will, increase since the United States Supreme Court overturned the landmark ruling of *Roe v. Wade*, following the *Dobbs v. Jackson Women's Health Organization* of 2022. Following this ruling, many states enacted laws restricting access to abortion care. In many of these states, not only are the laws vague, but many also carry penalties of prison time for Ob/Gyns who perform abortive procedures. Given this dilemma, while there is currently limited data, anecdotal evidence reflects a trend of obstetrics and gynecology care providers relocating from states with restrictive policies to those without punitive laws, where evidence-based medicine remains the standard of care. As a result, the closure of hospitals and/or labor and delivery units across the country will further exacerbate healthcare deserts, increase disparities in access to evidence-based medical care, and exacerbate the poor health outcomes already plaguing the restricting states, including and probably increasing the risk of postpartum hemorrhage, its associated complications, and the maternal mortality rate [16, 31].

Uninsured and underinsured persons face significant barriers to accessing adequate medical care [33, 34]. Many of the abortion-restricted state legislatures had also previously declined the increased Medicaid eligibility that was offered under the American Restrictive Rescue Plan Act of 2021, which, in conjunction with the overturning of Roe v. Wade, further inhibited access to care in many underserved areas. Consequently, these states had increased rates of pregnancy complications, as well as increased maternal and infant mortality [16].

7.2 Systems-related factor 2: Structure

The second systems-related factor that contributes to quality care in the setting of PPH is structure [32]. If a hospital does not have the equipment or medications needed to treat hemorrhage effectively, obviously, the quality of the care is going to be inhibited [32]. Protocols for managing postpartum hemorrhage should be established, and obstetric care teams must be thoroughly trained and proficient in these protocols to ensure the efficient delivery of care [32].

7.3 Systems-related factor 3: Blood loss estimation

The third factor contributing to lapses in quality care is the process of estimating blood loss [32]. Multiple studies have shown that providers do not accurately predict blood loss during a delivery [32]. It is therefore prudent to have processes in place to ensure accurate estimation of this metric in order to facilitate the initiation of PPH protocols when appropriate. The implementation of quantitative blood loss (QBL) in lieu of estimated blood loss in the obstetric setting can reduce the over- or under-estimation of blood loss and contribute to the timely management of postpartum hemorrhage [32].

8. The role of racial inequalities

In addition to system-related factors, racial inequalities, as well as implicit and explicit bias, have been identified as directly contributing to an increased incidence of PPH, which subsequently contributes to disparities in maternal morbidity and mortality in the United States [4, 35–37]. The evidence is abundant and clear that Caucasian women are less likely to experience postpartum hemorrhage than African Americans, Asians, and Native Hawaiians and other Pacific Islanders, but are more likely to receive blood transfusions [4]. In the United States, compared to white persons, adverse postpartum hemorrhage outcomes are increased in persons of color, regardless of level of education, employment status, or income [4, 38–40]. African Americans, when they do experience PPH secondary to uterine atony, are more likely to undergo invasive interventions, including hysterectomy [4, 36]. It is often underserved communities that live in maternity care deserts and have a lack of reliable insurance, further augmenting their risk of poor health outcomes. As a nation, the United States must address the systemic, racial, and logistical root causes of maternal mortality in order to decrease the appalling morbidity and mortality rates faced by our population. Prioritizing efforts to reduce the incidence and sequelae of postpartum hemorrhage should be a central focus in this process. Otherwise, the United States will continue to produce maternal health metrics similar to developing nations and never improve the healthcare system to be on par with, or better than, that of other developed nations.

Author details

Rebecca Bradley[1] and Alexander Juusela[2*]

1 Christus St. Michael Hospital, Texarkana, TX, United States of America

2 Newark Beth Israel Medical Center, Newark, NJ, United States of America

*Address all correspondence to: alex.l.juusela@gmail.com

References

[1] Fleszar LG, Bryant AS, Johnson CO, Blacker BF, Aravkin A, Baumann M, et al. Trends in state-level maternal mortality by racial and ethnic group in the United States. Journal of the American Medical Association. 2023;**330**(1):52-61. DOI: 10.1001/jama.2023.9043

[2] Hoyert DL. Maternal Mortality Rates in the United States. Atlanta, USA: Centers for Disease Control and Prevention; 2022. Available from: https://www.cdc.gov/nchs/data/hestat/maternal-mortality/2022/maternal-mortality-rates-2022.pdf [Accessed: August 10, 2024]

[3] Escobar MF, Nassar AH, Theron G, Barnea ER, Nicholson W, Ramasauskaite D, et al. FIGO recommendations on the management of postpartum hemorrhage 2022. International Journal of Gynaecology and Obstetrics. 2022;**157**(Suppl 1):3-50. DOI: 10.1002/ijgo.14116

[4] Okunlola O, Raza S, Osasan S, Sethia S, Batool T, Bambhroliya Z, et al. Race/ethnicity as a risk factor in the development of postpartum hemorrhage: A thorough systematic review of disparity in the relationship between pregnancy and the rate of postpartum hemorrhage. Cureus. 2022;**14**(6):e26460. DOI: 10.7759/cureus.26460

[5] Treml AB, Gorlin JB, Dutton RP, Scavone BM. Massive transfusion protocols: A survey of academic medical centers in the United States. Anesthesia & Analgesia. 2017;**124**(1):277-281. DOI: 10.1213/ANE.0000000000001610

[6] Bienstock JL, Eke AC, Hueppchen NA. Postpartum hemorrhage. The New England Journal of Medicine. 2021;**384**(17):1635-1645. DOI: 10.1056/NEJMra1513247

[7] Anderson JM, Etches D. Prevention and management of postpartum hemorrhage. American Family Physician. 2007;**75**(6):875-882

[8] Sheldon W, Blum J, Vogel J, Souza J, Gülmezoglu A, Winikoff B. Postpartum haemorrhage management, risks, and maternal outcomes: Findings from the World Health Organization multicountry survey on maternal and newborn health. BJOG: An International Journal of Obstetrics & Gynaecology. 2014;**121**: 5-13. DOI: 10.1111/1471-0528.12636

[9] Koutras A, Fasoulakis Z, Syllaios A, Garmpis N, Diakosavvas M, Pagkalos A, et al. Physiology and pathology of contractility of the myometrium. In Vivo. 2021;**35**(3):1401-1408. DOI: 10.21873/invivo.12392. Epub 2021 Apr 28

[10] Coad SL, Dahlgren LS, Hutcheon JA. Risks and consequences of puerperal uterine inversion in the United States, 2004 through 2013. American Journal of Obstetrics and Gynecology. 2017;**217**(3):377.e1-377.e6. DOI: 10.1016/j.ajog.2017.05.018. Epub 2017 May 15

[11] Einerson BD, Gilner JB, Zuckerwise LC. Placenta accreta spectrum. Obstetrics & Gynecology. 2023;**142**(1):31-50. DOI: 10.1097/AOG.0000000000005229

[12] Macones G, A, Peipert J, Nelson DB, Odibo A, Stevens EJ, Stamilio DM, et al. Maternal complications with vaginal birth after cesarean delivery: A multicenter study. American Journal of Obstetrics and Gynecology. 2005;**193**(5):1656-1662

[13] Anaposala S, Kalluru PKR, Calderon Martinez E, Bhavanthi S, Gundoji CR. Postpartum hemorrhage and tranexamic acid: A literature review. Cureus. 2023;**15**(5):e38736. DOI: 10.7759/cureus.38736

[14] Jackson KW, Allbert JR, Schemmer GK, Elliot M, Humphrey A, Taylor J. A randomized controlled trial comparing oxytocin administration before and after placental delivery in the prevention of postpartum hemorrhage. American Journal of Obstetrics and Gynecology. 2001;**185**(4):873-877. DOI: 10.1067/mob.2001.117363

[15] Koch DM, Rattmann YD. Use of misoprostol in the treatment of postpartum hemorrhage: A pharmacoepidemiological approach. Einstein (Sao Paulo). 2019;**18**:eAO5029. DOI: 10.31744/einstein_journal/2020AO5029

[16] Declercq E et al. The U.S. maternal health divide: The limited maternal health services and worse outcomes of states proposing new abortion restrictions. Commonwealth Fund. 2022;**2**(2):10.26099/z7dz-8211

[17] Mhyre JM, Shilkrut A, Kuklina EV, Callaghan WM, Creanga AA, Kaminsky S, et al. Massive blood transfusion during hospitalization for delivery in New York State, 1998-2007. Obstetrics and Gynecology. 2013;**122**(6):1288-1294. DOI: 10.1097/AOG.0000000000000021

[18] Vogel JP, Nguyen PY, Ramson J, De Silva MS, Pham MD, Sultana S, et al. Effectiveness of care bundles for prevention and treatment of postpartum hemorrhage: A systematic review. American Journal of Obstetrics and Gynecology. 2024;**231**(1):67-91. DOI: 10.1016/j.ajog.2024.01.012. Epub 2024 Feb 7

[19] D'Alton ME, Rood KM, Smid MC, Simhan HN, Skupski DW, Subramaniam A, et al. Intrauterine vacuum-induced hemorrhage-control device for rapid treatment of postpartum hemorrhage. Obstetrics and Gynecology. 2020;**136**(5):882-891. DOI: 10.1097/AOG.0000000000004138

[20] Walfish M et al. Maternal haemorrhage. British Journal of Anesthesia. 2009;**103**(suppl. 1):i43-i57

[21] Alves ÁLL, Nagahama G, Nozaki AM. Surgical management of postpartum hemorrhage. Revista Brasileira de Ginecologia e Obstetrícia/ RBGO Gynecology and Obstetrics (Thieme Revinter Publicações Ltda). Oct 2020;**42**(10):679-686. EN. 2020/10/31. DOI: 10.1055/s-0040-1719159. Available from: http://www.thieme-connect.com/products/ejournals/abstract/10.1055/s-0040-1719159

[22] Guasch E, Gilsanz F. Massive obstetric hemorrhage: Current approach to management. Medicine Intensiva (English Edition). 2016;**40**:298-310

[23] Tsirulnikov MS. Ligation of the uterine vessels during obstetrical hemorrhages. Immediate and long-term results (author's transl). Journal de Gynecologie, Obstetrique et Biologie de la Reproduction. 1979;**8**:751-753

[24] AbdRabbo SA. Stepwise uterine devascularization: A novel technique for management of uncontrolled postpartum hemorrhage with preservation of the uterus. American Journal of Obstetrics and Gynecology. 1994;**171**:694-700

[25] Quenu E, Duval P. Bilateral ligation of the hypogastric artery by transperitoneal approach. Revue de Chirurgie. 1898;**18**:979-992

[26] Doumouchtsis SK, Papageorghiou AT, Arulkumaran S.

Systematic review of conservative management of postpartum hemorrhage: What to do when medical treatment fails. Obstetrical & Gynecological Survey. 2007;**62**(8):540-547. DOI: 10.1097/01.ogx.0000271137.81361.93

[27] Thakur M, Thakur A. Uterine inversion. In: StatPearls. Treasure Island (FL): StatPearls Publishing; 2024. Available from: https://www.ncbi.nlm.nih.gov/books/NBK525971/

[28] James AH, McLintock C, Lockhart E. Postpartum hemorrhage: When uterotonics and sutures fail. American Journal of Hematology. 2012;**87**(S1):S16-S22. DOI: 10.1002/ajh.23156

[29] McLintock C. Prevention and treatment of postpartum hemorrhage: Focus on hematological aspects of management. Program Hematology: The American Society of Hematology Education. 2020;**2020**(1):542. DOI: 10.1182/hematology.2020000139

[30] Erez O, Othman M, Rabinovich A, Leron E, Gotsch F, Thachil J. DIC in pregnancy – Pathophysiology, clinical characteristics, diagnostic scores, and treatments. Journal of Blood Medicine. 2022;**13**:21. DOI: 10.2147/JBM.S273047

[31] Markus AR, Pillai D. Mapping the location of health centers in relation to "maternity care deserts": Associations with utilization of women's health providers and services. Medical Care. 2021;**59**(Suppl 5):S434-S440. DOI: 10.1097/MLR.0000000000001611

[32] Federspiel JJ, Eke AC, Eppes CS. Postpartum hemorrhage protocols and benchmarks: Improving care through standardization. American Journal of Obstetrics & Gynecology MFM. 2023;**5**(2S):100740. DOI: 10.1016/j.ajogmf.2022.100740.Epub 2022 Sep 2

[33] Fontenot J, Brigance C, Lucas R, Stoneburner A. Navigating geographical disparities: Access to obstetric hospitals in maternity care deserts and across the United States. BMC Pregnancy and Childbirth. 2024;**24**(1):350. DOI: 10.1186/s12884-024-06535-7

[34] Hofmeyr GJ, Abdel-Aleem H, Abdel-Aleem MA. Uterine massage for preventing postpartum haemorrhage. Cochrane Database Syst Rev. 2013;(7):CD006431. DOI: 10.1002/14651858.CD006431.pub3

[35] Wetta LA, Szychowski JM, Seals S, Mancuso MS, Biggio JR, Tita AT. Risk factors for uterine atony/postpartum hemorrhage requiring treatment after vaginal delivery. American Journal of Obstetrics and Gynecology. 2013;**209**(1):51.e1-51.e6. DOI: 10.1016/j.ajog.2013.03.011. Epub 2013 Mar 15

[36] Gyamfi-Bannerman C, Srinivas SK, Wright JD, Goffman D, Siddiq Z, D'Alton ME, et al. Postpartum hemorrhage outcomes and race. American Journal of Obstetrics and Gynecology. 2018;**219**(2):185.e1-185.e10. DOI: 10.1016/j.ajog.2018.04.052. Epub 2018 May 9

[37] Mujahid MS, Kan P, Leonard SA, Hailu EM, Wall-Wieler E, Abrams B, et al. Birth hospital and racial and ethnic differences in severe maternal morbidity in the state of California. American Journal of Obstetrics and Gynecology. 2021;**224**(2):219.e1-219.e15. DOI: 10.1016/j.ajog.2020.08.017. Epub 2020 Aug 13

[38] Bisson C, Dautel S, Patel E, Rana S. Maternal mortality in the United States: The pervasive effects of racism. Med. 2022;**3**(6):361-364. DOI: 10.1016/j.medj.2022.05.008

[39] Howell EA. Reducing disparities in severe maternal morbidity and mortality. Clinical Obstetrics and Gynecology. 2018;**61**(2):387-399. DOI: 10.1097/GRF.0000000000000349

[40] Petersen EE, Davis NL, Goodman D, Cox S, Syverson C, Seed K, et al. Racial/ethnic disparities in pregnancy-related deaths - United States, 2007-2016. MMWR. Morbidity and Mortality Weekly Report. 2019;**68**(35):762-765. DOI: 10.15585/mmwr.mm6835a3

Chapter 8

Operative Vaginal Delivery (OVD) in Contemporary Obstetrics

Benjamin Joseph Nggada

Abstract

In contemporary obstetrics, operative vaginal delivery still plays a key role in reducing morbidity and improving fetal outcomes and has proven to be inversely proportional to caesarean delivery rates. Therefore, in settings where the rate of instrumental vaginal delivery is high, the caesarean delivery rate is proportionally lower. The dwindling incidence of instrumental vaginal delivery is attributed to the lack of skills accusation, modification of medical curriculum, increased caesarean section rate, and increased litigation in contemporary practice. In the hands of a skilled operator when all parameters are met, the forceps or vacuum is a masterpiece and valuable tool in expediting the delivery of the fetus with resultant improved neonatal outcome.

Keywords: vacuum extraction, forceps delivery, prolonged second stage, caesarean delivery, assisted vaginal delivery, vacuum-assisted birth, deep impacted fetal head

1. Introduction

The use of devices to expedite vaginal delivery with or without maternal effort is considered as operative vaginal delivery (OVD). These devices and/or instruments are the popular forceps and vacuum [1]. The increased gain in knowledge and innovation towards operative vaginal birth has led to the production of newer devices like the Odon vacuum device [2], modifications of the Pro-Nata Yorkshire operative forceps and kiwi vacuum devices, which are now available in the market and attest to the gain in knowledge and innovation towards instrumental vaginal delivery [3, 4].

The term OVD has been used interchangeably with instrumental vaginal delivery, operative vaginal birth, or assisted vaginal delivery. In contemporary obstetrics, OVD still plays a key role in reducing morbidity and improving fetal outcomes and has been proven to be inversely proportional to caesarean delivery rates [1, 5–7]. Consequently, in health care settings where the rate of OVD is high, the rate of abdominal delivery is inversely proportional [1]. The dwindling incidence of OVD is attributable to diminished skills, modification of medical curriculum, increased acceptability of caesarean delivery, and hostile litigation climate in contemporary practice [8–10]. When all parameters are met, in the hands of a skilled operator the forceps or vacuum is a masterpiece and valuable tool in expediting the delivery of the fetus with resultant improved neonatal outcome [1].

2. History lane

It has been documented that there are more than 700 varieties of obstetric forceps that date back to 1500 BC since the idea of operative vaginal delivery was conceived [7]. The writings of Hippocrates attest to some form of operative vaginal birth between 500 BC and 500 AD and Hindu medicine has described these obstetric skills since the sixth century BC [11]. The purpose of forceps-assisted delivery was to prevent morbidities among mothers and newborns. The field of obstetrics and "man-midwifery" was brought to the limelight by the Chamberlen brothers [7, 11]. Peter the Elder and Peter the Younger are two sons of French Huguenot William Chamberlen who escaped to England in the sixth century due to prosecution and served as Queen's surgeon. Peter the Younger continued the family tradition of midwifery and forceps delivery [5, 11, 12]. Francois Mauriceau challenged Huguenot Williams when he wanted to sell his secret in 1670 to the French government and demanded that he deliver a 38-year-old rachitic dwarf [11]. Although the first Chamberlen tools were found in 1813, forceps replicas first appeared in the early 1700s [11]. To prevent child loss and complications of forceps delivery, the pelvic curvature and the "English lock" were created by William Smellie, and his work was published in the "Treatise on the Theory and Practice of Midwifery" released by him in 1752. His innovation and work was vehemently opposed by Elizabeth Nihell [11].

The beginning of vacuum extraction was described by James Yonge who initially described a hoover in 1705. This was made popular by Malmstrom in Europe [12, 13]. A disproportionate increase in vacuum deliveries compared to forceps has gradually become the trend in operative vaginal birth over the years. These have been the result of concerns generated over the years of associated complications, lack of proper training, increased litigations, and concerns for the safety of the mother and her newborn [13].

3. Updated data

The rate of operative vaginal birth depends on several factors which vary in hospitals and different regions of the world. While it is the belief that the trend is on the decline, the rates are high in developed countries compared to developing countries [1]. In the UK, the rate of instrumental vaginal delivery has been quoted to range between 10% and 15% [14]. The rate appears to vary across Europe, with a reported low incidence of 1.4% in Croatia and 14.4% in Spain following a survey done in 2019 [15, 16]. In the United States, trends in operative vaginal birth showed a pattern of decline in a population-based study with an incident rate of 5.9%. Vacuum-assisted delivery was 4.8% and forceps was 1.1% with a decline of 5.8 and 4.1%, respectively, between 2005 and 2013 [17]. In a recent expert review by Bahl et al. over three decades in the United States, caesarean delivery has steadily increased and hovers above 30% while Vacuum deliveries are below 5% and forceps delivery is almost nonexistent (**Figure 1**) [1].

The decline in the rate of operative vaginal birth is more profound in middle- and low-income countries. In an institutional review of operative vaginal birth in South Africa between 2005 and 2019 in two academic hospitals, Dutywa et al. reported an incidence of 1.36 and 1.60%, respectively, and a decline was noted to be over 9% in both institutions. The downward trend of instrumental deliveries might be attributed to a lack of training and other barriers that needed to be identified [18]. A pooled

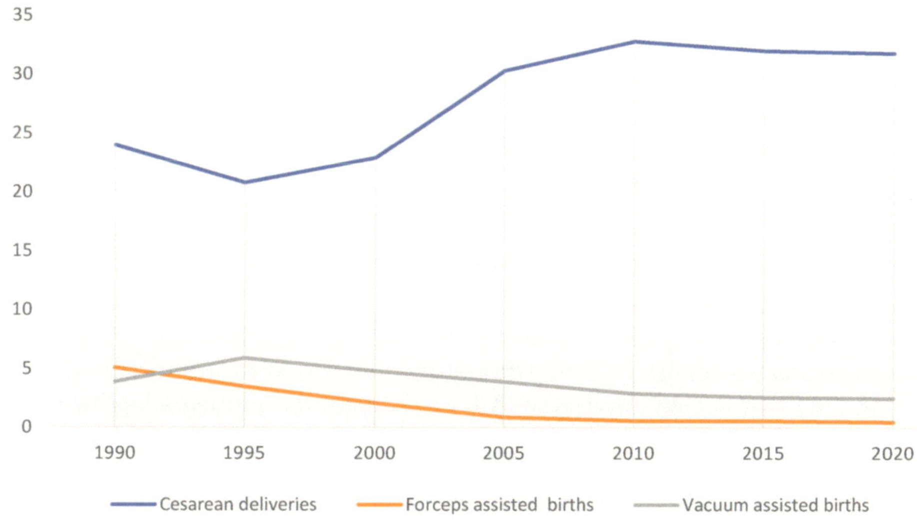

Figure 1.
Comparison and trend of operative vaginal delivery and caesarean section.

prevalence of 7.98% operative vaginal delivery in Sub-Saharan Africa was documented following a systematic review and meta-analysis. However, such a rate might be sampled from institutions with higher rates of OVD [19]. In examining the declining trend of operative vaginal deliveries in Nigeria, Anozie and co-authors surveyed Obstetricians and Gynaecologists and unravelled the reasons for the decline in this practice. Lack of instruments, skills, and department protocols was highlighted. The increased rate of litigation, the safety of caesarean deliveries, and patient preference have significantly decreased the incidence of instrumental deliveries [9].

4. Role of instrumental delivery in contemporary obstetrics

The complexity of the second stage of labour and options of delivery in the event of the need to expedite the delivery will continue to intrigue health workers in women's health. The aim is not always to achieve a vaginal birth but to have an outcome with little or no morbidity to the mother and her neonate(s). However, most deliveries at full cervical dilatation or the advanced first stage of labour are complicated. Particularly, a caesarean section in the second stage of labour has been associated with higher morbidity to the mother and newborn with a higher rate of special care admission compared to a successful OVD [1, 20]. The second stage caesarean section has been associated with major risks of obstetric haemorrhage, genital tract trauma, maternal dissatisfaction, prolonged hospitalisation, and increased risk of neonatal trauma [20]. The decision delivery interval is relatively faster when the route of instrumental delivery is preferred compared to caesarean delivery and this is particularly helpful in developing countries where the decision delivery interval is agonisingly longer with abysmal emergency preparedness and response rate with associated complications compared to high-income countries [20].

An argument in favour of OVD is the better understanding of the mechanism(s) of labour and the ability to use 3D models, imaging modalities, and artificial intelligence to predict delivery outcomes in advanced labour and the advent of newer instruments with safety mechanisms [21, 22]. Newer and safer innovations have been recently incorporated in women's health practice which is less traumatic and also can give the operative feedback during traction. The Pro-Nata Yorkshire operative forceps have been invited to be safe, and the handheld Kiwi vacuum and the Odon device are a testament that OVD will continue to have its rightful place in contemporary obstetrics [1, 2, 23, 24].

5. The instruments

The instruments are designed to partially or wholly assist the woman in vaginal birth [1]. Modification has occurred over several decades to improve adapting the pelvic architecture for vacuum and improve cup efficiency, resulting in less trauma to the mother and her fetal scalp and skull for vacuum devices [24, 25]. Several forceps were developed for different purposes, but the anatomy of these forceps are similar [5, 12]. Forceps essentially have four major components, which are the handles, locks, shanks, and blades. The base of the forceps consists of the handles, followed by the lock, then the shanks, and lastly, the blade. The blades are described in a fashion to represent the foot which has a heel closer to the shanks and a toe at the tip of the blade [5]. The blade has two curves: the inner aspect of the blade has the cephalic curve while the outer is the pelvic curve. The blade can either be solid or closed, open, or fenestrated, while the shanks can be overlapping, separated, or parallel [5, 26]. The Eillot/Tucker-McLane forceps are overlapping and can easily be remembered with the phrase "Tucker tucked in" while the Simpson and the Wrigley forceps have

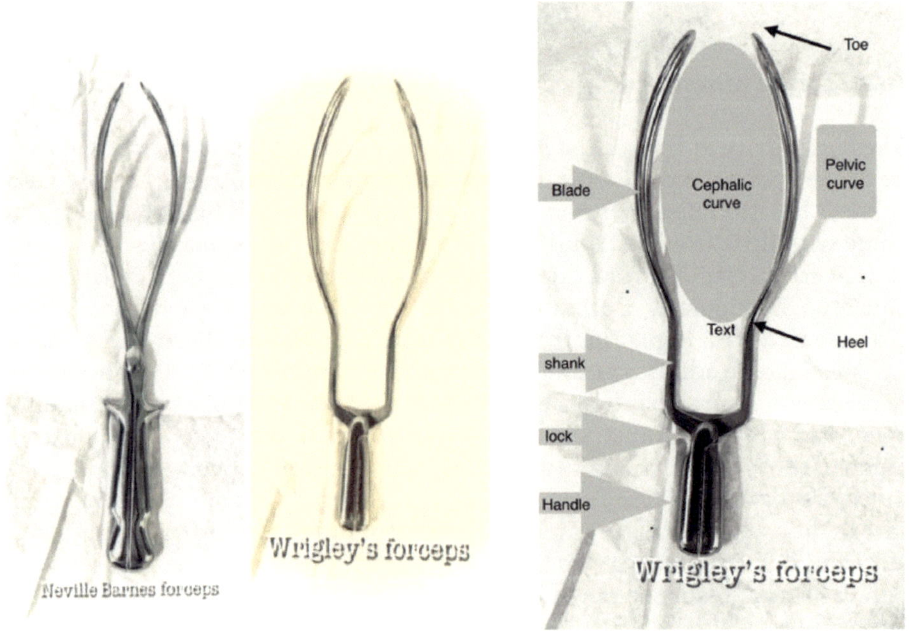

Figure 2.
Forceps.

shanks that are separated which can be remembered by the phrase "Simpson shanks separated". The Kielland forceps are specially designed for rotational manoeuvres due to the slight reverse pelvic curvature and a sliding lock which is suitable for correction of asynclitism. The piper forceps have the unique characteristics of a reverse pelvic curvature with the shanks tilted downwards, which is suitable for stabilisation and delivery of the after-coming head in breech presentation (**Figure 2**) [26].

The popular Kiwi vacuum is a handheld device developed in 1990 by Aldo Vacca [27] compared to the conventional vacuum developed by Malmstrom in 1957, which has a bulky suction machine attached to it [27, 28]. The innovation of Kiwi vacuum has been further developed by Laborie Medical Technologies Corp to a complete vacuum delivery system that has Omnicup, Omni-MT, Omni-C, and the Procup. The Omni-MT has a traction force indicator and is considered versatile while the Omni-C is particularly designed for delivery at caesarean section (this is not technically considered instrumental vaginal delivery) and the Procup is a soft cup for low occipital anterior and outlet delivery (**Table 1**) [30]. See **Figure 3**.

Cups	Indication(s)	Types
Soft	Outlet and low occipito-anterior <45°	• Kiwi ProCup and Kiwi Omni cup • Silc, Gentle Vac, and secure cups • Silastic, Reusable and Vac-U-Nate cups • Standard MityVac Cup and Soft Touch cups
Rigid	Anterior cups – outlet and low occipito-anterior <45°	• M-Style MityVac cup • Flex cup • Malmstrom, Bird and O'Neil cups
Rigid	Posterior cups- occipito-anterior >45, occipito-posterior and Occipito-Transverse	• Kiwi OmniCup • M-Style MityVac cup • Malmstrom, Bird and O'Neil cups
Adapted from: Ref. [29]		

Table 1.
Vacuum delivery cups: classification and use.

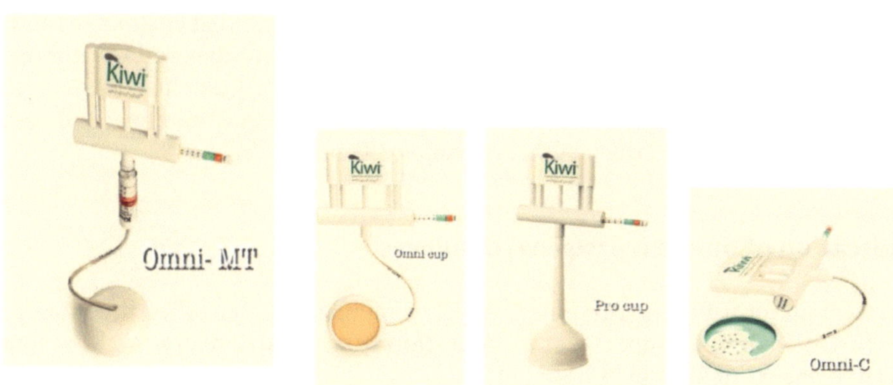

Figure 3.
Kiwi vacuum system.

Full abdominal and vaginal examination
• The fetal head is ≤1/5 palpable per abdomen (in most cases not palpable) • The cervix is fully dilated, and the membranes ruptured • The Station is at the level of ischial spines or below • The position of the fetal head has been determined • Caput and moulding are no more than moderate • The pelvis is deemed adequate
Preparation of mother
• Clear explanation given and informed consent taken and documented in women's case notes • Trust was established and full cooperation was sought and agreed upon with the woman • Appropriate analgesia is in place: for mid-pelvic or rotational birth, this will usually be a regional block; a pudendal block may be acceptable depending on urgency; and a perineal block may be sufficient for low or outlet birth • The maternal bladder has been emptied • The indwelling catheter has been removed or the balloon deflated • Aseptic technique
Preparation of staff
• The operator has the knowledge, experience and skills necessary • Adequate facilities are available (equipment, bed, lighting) and access to an operating theatre • Backup plan: for mid-pelvic births, theatre facilities should be available to allow a caesarean birth to be performed without delay; A senior obstetrician should be present if an inexperienced obstetrician is conducting the birth • Anticipation of complications that may arise (e.g. shoulder dystocia, perineal trauma, postpartum haemorrhage) • Personnel present who are trained in neonatal resuscitation
Adapted from: RCOG green top guideline. Murphy et al. [20].

Table 2.
Prerequisites for OVD.

6. Prerequisites for OVD – RCOG criteria

Adhering to and using the prerequisites for OVD as a checklist ensures success and minimises the likelihood of failure and morbidities for the mother and her unborn fetus. The royal college of Obstetricians and Gynaecologists' guidelines on assisted vaginal birth grouped the safety criteria into three categories: Abdominal and vaginal findings, the mother, and the healthcare worker (**Table 2**) [14].

7. Indication of operative vaginal delivery

Indication for using instruments to assist in vaginal delivery, when the prerequisites are met and there are no contraindications to vaginal delivery, could be fetal, maternal, or a combination of both [14].

The indication should be discussed by the managing team and the mother should be involved. Consent should be obtained as per local department protocol and documented (**Table 3**).

Fetal
Suspected fetal compromise (cardiotocography pathological, abnormal fetal blood sampling result, thick meconium)
Maternal
Nulliparous women – lack of continuing progress for 3 hours (total of active and passive second-stage labour) with regional analgesia or 2 hours without regional analgesia
Parous women – lack of continuing progress for 2 hours (total of active and passive second-stage labour) with regional analgesia or 1 hour without regional analgesia
Maternal exhaustion or distress
Medical indications to avoid Valsalva manoeuvre
Combined
Fetal and maternal indications for assisted vaginal birth often coexist.
Adapted from RCOG green top guideline. Murphy et al. [20].

Table 3.
Indication for OVD in contemporary obstetrics practice.

8. Contraindication to OVD

When vaginal delivery is not feasible or delivery via the vaginal route could result in an increase in morbidity to the mother and her fetus, then instrumental delivery should not be attempted under any circumstances. Other relative contraindications are fetal bleeding disorders whether diagnosed or suspected (alloimmune thrombocytopenia), increased risk of fracture (osteogenesis imperfecta), and gestational age less than 32 weeks because of increased tendencies for the babies to develop cephalohematoma [1, 14]. The risk of subgaleal haemorrhage between 32 and 36 weeks is substantially high in a retrospective survey of over 5000 women [14, 31]. Therefore, the use of OVD should be done with caution in women with foetuses within the gestational age bracket. Blood-borne viral infection in the mother is not an absolute contraindication to OVD. However, where there is an increased risk of scalp trauma or abrasion, OVD should be avoided [14]. OVD should only be attempted in a woman who is fully dilated. Inability to precisely determine the vertex position and when the vertex is above the ischial spine is an absolute contraindication in contemporary practice [1]. The author strongly believes that lack of proficiency in OVD by the healthcare worker is an absolute contraindication to OVD.

9. Training in OVD, advocacy for training, and the role of artificial intelligence

The dwindling rate of OVD has been attributed to several factors, however, one factor that has been consistent in most reviews and surveys is the exponential drop in training and teaching to postgraduate medical residents and the lack of passion to pass this long tradition to the future generation of physicians in women's health [1, 5, 9, 32]. Right, effective, and adequate training is the key to reviving the art and science of OVD. Simulation is safe and effective [32]. Additionally, clinical mentorship from experts and physicians with a passion for OVD and supportive supervision is key to transmitting knowledge and skills of OVD [33]. To advocate for OVD, more research is needed to bridge the knowledge gap in evidence, technical expert view, and women's views, as recommended by the WHO technical brief on assisted vaginal birth [34]. Training institutions and societies in women's health need to come up with a consensus training guide and manual that is acceptable for all. Ultrasound in labour has been promised to improve outcomes by precisely determining the descent of the presenting part and pinpointing the location of the position of the head [35, 36]. Gradually incorporating artificial intelligence into obstetrics and its role in predicting mode of delivery has been seen to outperform traditional methods [37, 38]. The unmet research gap in OVD with AI is huge and can be a game changer in the near future.

10. Classification of OVD

The classification of OVD determines the instrument to be used, the competency level needed for the delivery and helps with proper communication between the patient and the managing team. The classification below is from the patient and safety quality committee of the Society of Maternal-Fetal Medicine (SMFM) (**Table 4**) [39].

11. Procedure and documentation

Operative vaginal deliveries require the skills and competence to increase the likelihood of success and reduce potential morbidities to the mother and her baby. Ideally, a checklist should be used to improve outcomes and ensure quality assurance and patient safety (**Figure 4**) [39].

SMFM OVD checklist.

An OVD should have the following considerations according to the SMFM OVD checklist [39].

Outlet
1. Scalp visible at the introitus without separating the labia
2. Fetal skull at the pelvic floor
3. Fetal head at or on the perineum
4. Sagittal suture in anteroposterior diameter or right or left occiput-anterior or posterior position
5. Rotation 45 degrees or less
Low forceps
1. The leading point of the fetal skull at station +2 cm or more and not on the pelvic floor
2. Without rotation: Rotation 45 degrees or less (right or left occiput anterior to occiput anterior, or right or left occiput posterior to occiput posterior)
3. With rotation: rotation is greater than 45 degrees
Mid forceps
1. Station above +2 cm but head engaged

Adapted from: Ref. [39].

Table 4.
Classification of OVD.

Operative Vaginal Delivery: Checklist for Preparation and Performance
SAMPLE VERSION: Should be modified to fit requirements of local institution

Preparation and Prerequisites
- ☐ What is the primary indication for operative delivery?
  - o Prolonged second stage
  - o Fetal compromise (suspected or potential)
  - o Maternal benefit (such as medical problem or exhaustion)
- ☐ Is the estimated fetal weight reasonable for vaginal delivery? Record weight________ g
- ☐ Is the cervix fully dilated and retracted?
- ☐ Are the maternal pelvis dimensions judged to be adequate for vaginal delivery?
- ☐ Is the fetal head is engaged? Record station ___________
- ☐ Is the fetal head position known (for example, occiput anterior) Record position___________
- ☐ Are the fetal membranes ruptured?
- ☐ Is there a known or suspected fetal contraindication (for example, thrombocytopenia, hemophilia, von Willebrand disease, osteogenesis imperfecta)?
- ☐ Have benefits and risks been discussed with patient and has she agreed to the procedure?
- ☐ Where should procedure be performed (delivery room or operating room)?
- ☐ Have the following people been notified?
  - o L&D nursing staff (charge nurse, others as needed)
  - o Obstetrics attending (if procedure to be performed by trainee)
  - o Anesthesiology
  - o Pediatrics (NICU, pediatrician, or neonatal team)

Pre-Procedure Time Out
- ☐ Are all team members present (OB, nursing, anesthesia, pediatrics)?
- ☐ Does the patient identity match the chart?
- ☐ Will vacuum extraction be performed?
  - o Is gestational age at least 34 weeks?
  - o What pressure will be used?
  - o Will we follow our usual stopping rules (stop if 3 pop-offs, stop if not making progress with each pull, stop after 15 minutes, no changing to forceps if vacuum unsuccessful)
- ☐ Will forceps delivery be performed?
  - o Will we follow our usual stopping rules (stop if not making progress with each pull, stop after 15 minutes, no changing to vacuum if forceps unsuccessful)?
- ☐ Are contingencies in place for cesarean delivery if vaginal delivery is unsuccessful?
- ☐ Is anesthesia adequate for the procedure?
- ☐ Has the patient's bladder been emptied?
- ☐ What will be the indications to perform episiotomy?
- ☐ What preparations have been made for possible postpartum hemorrhage?
- ☐ Will we give a prophylactic antibiotic after procedure?
- ☐ Record time of placement of instrument _________________

Figure 4.
SMFM special statement: operative vaginal delivery. Am J Obstet Gynecol 2020.

1. Discussion of risks and benefits and consent from the mother

2. Consideration of the appropriate site for the procedure

3. Appropriate team members present for delivery

4. Confirmation of patient identity

5. Detail of vacuum delivery (local guidelines should determine, e.g., vacuum use only from 34 weeks)

6. Details of forceps (standardised stopping rules)

7. Preparation for postpartum haemorrhage

8. Prophylactic antibiotics

11.1 Steps in performing a forceps delivery

Consider all initial steps highlighted in this chapter before the application of forceps and ensure informed consent is already in place (verbal consent is sufficient). Start by positioning the woman in a lithotomy position and stand or sit directly facing the perineum. A ghost application to articulate the forceps should be done to ensure that placement will be done in order [26]. For the left occiput-anterior position, hold the handle of the forceps with the fingertips of your left fingers and allow it to dangle perpendicularly to the ground [26, 40]. Use the tips of the index and the middle finger of the right hand to place them on the toe of the blade and the thumb on the heel of the blade with the palmer side of your hands [40]. Introduce the blade while the dorsum of your hand protects the vaginal wall. Guide the handle of the forceps down and push the blade mostly by the thumb on the heel of the blade. Repeat the same procedure on the right and ensure to articulate at the lock. Ensure that vaginal tissues are not trapped before traction is applied [26, 40]. Delivery of the head is done by applying traction. Horizontal traction is first applied with the right hand followed by a downward vertical pressure with the left hand which ensures flexion of the fetal head and maintains the axis of delivery to follow the pelvic curvature (Pajot's manoeuvre) [26, 40]. At the crowing of the head, which will be evident when the perineum is distended, a decision to evaluate and perform episiotomy to ease the perineal and soft tissue rigidity might be necessary at this point [26]. A lateral episiotomy is recommended at an angle of at least 60 degrees to the midline and it is advisable at the point that the perineum should be guarded which can be done by the assistant. The handle of the forceps can be elevated at this point in a J shape movement at the emergence of the posterior fontanelle below the symphysis pubis. This helps to mimic the natural cardinal movements of the mechanism of labour and to achieve extension of the fetal head [26]. The forceps blade can be dismantled once the fetal jaw is visible. The sequence is followed by restitution of the head and delivery of the shoulder to complete expulsion of the baby (**Figure 5**) [40].

11.2 Steps in performing a vacuum delivery

The principles of OPV are similar for both vacuum and forceps delivery. The location of the flexion point is crucial to the success of vacuum delivery because it helps to maintain and enhance the flexion of the head, thereby making the presenting diameter (smaller) favourable for vaginal delivery. There are four possibilities for placing the vacuum cup [4]:

1. Flexing median: 2–3 centimetres anterior to the posterior fontanelle at the midline or sagittal suture lines. THIS IS THE FLEXION POINT.

2. Flexing paramedian: 2–3 centimetres anterior to the posterior fontanelle, however, the cup is skewed lateral to one side either to the left or right, and not at the midline.

3. Deflexing median: The cup is placed at the midline or sagittal suture lines close to the anterior fontanelle.

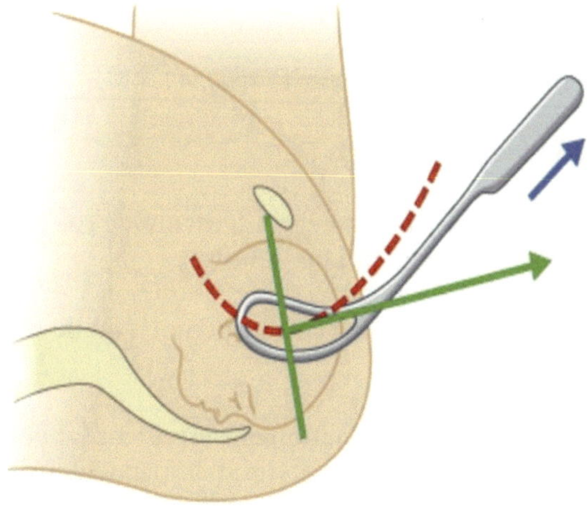

Figure 5.
Forceps traction for delivery (Pajot's manoeuvre).

4. Deflexing paramedian: The cup is placed close to the anterior fontanelle but skewed lateral to one side to the left or right.

These applications (2–4) present an unfavourable larger diameter to the pelvis with the tendency for more traction force, scalp trauma, and more likelihood of failure [4].

The precise position and synclitic orientation of the fetal head should be determined before the application of the vacuum cup. The steps for performing a vacuum OVD using the Kiwi Omni-MT are described below (**Figure 6**).

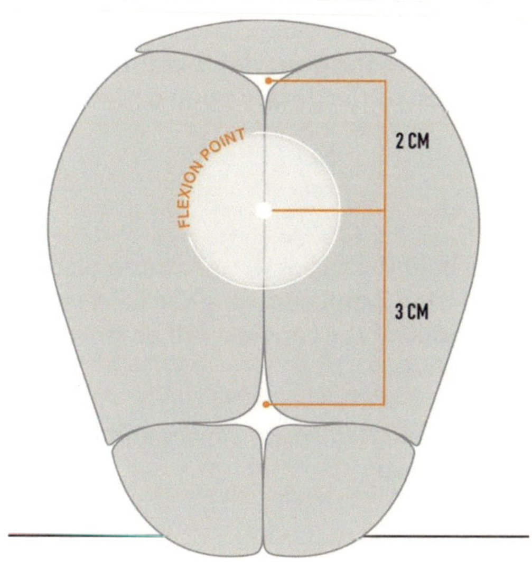

Figure 6.
The flexion point (Flexing median).

11.3 Aldo Vacca five-step technique

- Know your patient and create a rapport [4, 27, 41, 42].

- Evaluate for a valid indication of OVD.

- Communication should be patient-centred, involving the birth partner, health-care workers looking after her, and her family.

- Your skills are important (you must be competent), while trainees must be supervised.

- Conduct a thorough clinical examination of the patient (abdominal and vaginal examination). Detailed examination of the abdomen will include the number of fetuses, lie, presentation, attitude, and descent (the head should not be more than 1/5 palpable per abdomen). Check the fetal heart rate and review the cardiotocographic tracing. Vaginal assessment should include cervical dilatation, membranes must be ruptured, with the bladder emptied. The fetal position should be determined, caput and moulding should be assessed, and the anterior and posterior fontanelle should be evaluated to give an idea of the flexion point, degree of rotation, and synclitism. The descent and station must be determined, as well as extent of the fetal head descent during contractions; this is a contractions: this is a clue to envisage that delivery is possible. The colour of the liquor must be evaluated.

Step 1

- Measure the tip middle finger, the interphalangeal joint, and the metacarpal phalangeal joint and note them. (The vacuum stem has two marks at 6 and 11 cm).

- Locate the flexion point and calculate the compensation distance (put your middle finger on the posterior fontanelle and move 2–3 cm at the midline on the sagittal suture anterior to the posterior fontanelle and estimate the distance between the location of the flexion point and where your finger exits the introitus).

Step 2

- Insert the cup (Ideally hold the cup at the grove and place it at 12 o'clock position to determine if any rotation happens during the delivery. Avoid over-lubricating the cup and ensure the side of the cup that will be attached to the baby is as dry as possible).

- Use your non-examining hand to create a space and insert the cup sideways, then position it onto the fetal head.

- Step 3

Put your examining finger (middle) above the cup and slide the cup downward till you reach the compensation measurement. This will place the cup at the flexion point.

Step 4.

Create the vacuum till you reach 60 mmHg, the mark of the vacuum will guide you. Run your finger around the cup to exclude vaginal mucosa or any maternal tissue.

Step 5.

Apply traction during uterine contraction using a downward direction initially, then forward and upward movement (your thumb on the kiwi cup and the index finger on the fetal head. This helps to determine when the kiwi is separating and the likelihood of a pop-off and helps in determining if the head is descending. Traction should be synchronised with maternal contraction and traction should be stopped when there is no maternal contraction (this reduces the rate of pop-offs). At crowing, evaluate if an episiotomy is needed, which should be done at 60 degrees from the midline, and thereafter, manual perineum protection should be done. Once the baby's head is delivered then the vacuum pressure is released, and the shoulder and the rest of the body should be delivered subsequently.

11.4 When to abandon OVD?

It is prudent for any healthcare worker conducting an OVD to know when to abandon the procedure and opt for abdominal delivery. It will be catastrophic if that stop point is not recognised because there will be dire maternal fetal consequences which might often lead to litigation. A Vacuum-Assisted Birth (VAB) should be abandoned when there is evidence of no progressive descent during traction, and if three pulls do not bring the head to the perineum and there are two pop-offs despite correct application. Total application time should be less than 30 minutes. Any of these scenarios should be deemed appropriate to abandon VAB. There is an increased risk of complications, especially obstetric anal sphincter injuries, with the use of sequential instruments. Therefore, risk balancing should be considered regarding sequential instrument use or the alternative, which is an abdominal delivery. Forceps delivery should be discontinued when appears difficult to apply or articulate after application, especially if the handles become difficult to lock in. If rotation is not feasible or there is no eminent sign of delivery after three pulls, the procedure should be stopped [4, 10, 14, 39, 41, 42].

12. Complications

12.1 Management of impacted fetal head

An impacted fetal head and its sequalae is one of the complications that can occur after a failed OVD with several other complications following a successful OVD (**Table 5**). Therefore, whenever a decision is made for abdominal delivery after an attempted OVD, it should be considered a difficult caesarean section, and the most senior doctor or obstetrician should be at the delivery. The impacted fetal head can be relieved via manual vaginal disimpaction, the use of a fetal pillow, uterine relaxation, abdominal cephalic disimpaction, reverse breech extraction, and several Patwardhan techniques [48, 49].

13. Recommendations

In contemporary obstetrics, OVD will continue to play a critical role in women's health, especially in the management of the second stage of labour. While caesarean

Neonatal	
Complication	**Description**
Scalp effect	Visible marks of the cup attachment which are majorly of cosmetic concern with no clinical significance. This is transient and would resolve within days
Chignon	Artificial caput succedaneum is caused by the accumulation of interstitial fluid and microhemorrhages. It resolves between 12 and 18 hours
Scalp abrasion and laceration	No consensus in defining what scalp abrasion and lacerations are and what separates them. Correct cup placement and reducing pop-offs can reduce them. 10% in OVD
Retinal haemorrhage	More common in VAB. However, it is transient and has no associated long-term ophthalmological consequences. More common with vacuum and risk is 17–38%.
Neonatal jaundice	Appears more common in VAB compared to forceps. Treatment with phototherapy might be appropriate. Rates are quoted be to between 5 and 15% for OVD
Cephalohematoma	Accumulation of serosanguinous fluid under the periosteum of the fetal skull. The clinical implication is mild because the bleeding is limited in space and confined by the periosteum. 1–12% in VAB
Subgaleal haemorrhage	This is potentially life-threatening as a result of rupture of the emissary vessel that bleeds between the scalp and the aponeurosis and the periosteum of the fetal skull. Suture line does not limit its spread and neonates can present in shock because they can lose up to 80% of their blood volume. Predominant in VAB (3–6/1000)
Intracranial haemorrhage/ Intraventricular haemorrhage	Bleeding within the brain or in fluid space cavities of the brain of the newborn is said to be generally low but higher is said to be among babies born via VAB. Vacca, warns of the possibility of popping off at full traction as one of the causes. Rates are between 5 to 15% in 10,000
Facial nerve palsy	Rare in OVD and mainly occurs in forceps delivery
Skull fraction	Rare but possible. Reported to be between 1 in 664 in forceps and 1 in 860 in forceps-assisted delivery
Cervical spine injury	Mainly in high rotational forceps with Kielland which has been largely abandoned in contemporary practice. Rarely occur with a rate of 0.7/1000 rotational forceps
Fetal death	Extremely rare but possible
Maternal	
Vaginal hematomas/ Vulva hematoma	Vaginal tissue injuries are more likely to occur, and blunt trauma might result in microvascular injuries that can lead to hematoma formation
Urinary tract injuries	The proximity of the urethra meatus, urethra and bladder predisposes the urinary tract to injuries.
Anal sphincter injuries	Injury to the perineal muscles and anal sphincter complex. 1–4% for VAB and 8–12% for forceps delivery
Postpartum haemorrhage	Bleeding from common causes of PPH but higher tendencies from genital tract laceration (10–40%)

Table 5.
Vacuum-assisted birth and forceps delivery [14, 41–47].

section is an alternative, it might not be as swift as intended, with associated safety concerns and the increased risk of complications in a second-stage caesarean section should be considered. Relevant consensus training modules using the work of Aldo Vacca could be a strong foundation and a starting point for a training guide to OVD. Stakeholders including women should favour policies that will encourage training at institutions and provide the relevant equipment needed. Obstetricians should gradually incorporate artificial intelligence in predicting birth outcomes and the use of simulators will further enhance skill transfer and acquisition. Ultrasound in the second stage of labour will help to pinpoint the exact location of the fetal position and station with the possibility of improving the outcomes of OVD. Each obstetric unit should have regular training and conduct audits in OVD. There is a need for more research and innovation in the field of operative vaginal birth.

14. Conclusion

In the era of evidence-based medicine and technological advancement, the relevance of OVD is key to the management of the second stage of labour. Relevant training guides and mentorship from physicians who have the skills and passion to train and transfer skills will be a good strategy to keep the practice of OVD alive. A meticulous approach using a checklist and proper documentation of the procedure will fundamentally increase safety and reduce litigation from OVD.

Acknowledgements

Nurse/Midwife Nkungano Elijah for assisting with the pictures of the forceps used in this publication.

Author details

Benjamin Joseph Nggada
Division of Obstetrics and Gynaecology, Department of Maternal and Child Health, School of Medicine, University of Namibia, Namibia

*Address all correspondence to: bilyaminu@hotmail.com

References

[1] Bahl R, Hotton E, Crofts J, Draycott T. Assisted vaginal birth in the 21st century: Current practice and innovations. American Journal of Obstetrics and Gynecology. 2024;**230**:S917-S931. DOI: 10.1016/j.ajog.2022.12.305

[2] Hotton EJ, Alvarez M, Draycott TJ, Crofts JF, Hotton EJ, Lenguerrand E, et al. Outcomes of the novel Odon device in indicated operative vaginal birth. American Journal of Obstetrics and Gynecology. 2021;**224**(607):e1-607.e17. DOI: 10.1016/j.ajog.2020.12.017

[3] Deruelle P, Queste-Bothuyne E, Depret S, Subtil D. Five questions about the kiwi OmniCup™ vacuum extractor. Gynecologie Obstetrique et Fertilite. 2007;**35**(6):582-586

[4] Arulkumaran S. Malpresentation, malposition, cephalopelvic disproportion and obstetric procedures. In: Edmonds DK, editor. Dewhurst's Textbook of Obstetrics and Gynaecology. London UK: Blackwell Publishing; 2012. pp. 311-325

[5] Unuigbe J, Agbon-Ojeme G, Erhatiemwomon R, Maduako K. Instrumental vaginal deliveries: A review. Tropical Journal of Obstetrics and Gynaecology. 2018;**35**:99. DOI: 10.4103/tjog.tjog_49_18

[6] Government of Western Australia-North Metropolitan Health Services. Government of Western Australia-North Metropolitan Health Services. Subiaco, Western Australia: Operative Vaginal Delivery; 2023:1-16. Available from: https://www.kemh.health.wa.gov.au/~/media/HSPs/NMHS/Hospitals/WNHS/Documents/Clinical-guidelines/Obs-Gyn-Guidelines/Operative-Birth.pdf?thn=0

[7] Goetzinger KR, Macones GA. Operative vaginal delivery: Current trends in obstetrics. Women's Health. 2008;**4**:281-290. DOI: 10.2217/17455057.4.3.281

[8] Bailey PE. The disappearing art of instrumental delivery: Time to reverse the trend. International Journal of Gynecology & Obstetrics. 2005;**91**:89-96. DOI: 10.1016/j.ijgo.2005.05.016

[9] Anozie OB, Osaheni LL, Onu FA, Onoh RC, Ogah EO, Eze JN, et al. Declining rate of operative vaginal deliveries in Nigeria. Open Journal of Obstetrics and Gynecology. 2018;**08**:175-184. DOI: 10.4236/ojog.2018.83021

[10] Murphy DJ. Medico-legal considerations and operative vaginal delivery. Best Practice & Research. Clinical Obstetrics & Gynaecology. 2019;**56**:114-24. DOI: 10.1016/j.bpobgyn.2019.01.012

[11] Sheikh S, Ganesaratnam I, Jan H. The birth of forceps. JRSM Short Reports. 2013;**4**:1-4. DOI: 10.1177/2042533313478412

[12] Blackstone J, Katukuri V. Will vacuum delivery go the way of vaginal breech delivery. Contemporary OB/GYN. 2019;**64**(7):7-11

[13] Ali UA, Norwitz ER. Vacuum-Assisted Vaginal Delivery. Rev Obstet Gynecol. 2009;**2**(1):5-17

[14] Murphy DJ, Strachan BK, Bahl R. Assisted vaginal birth: Green-top guideline No. 26. BJOG: An International Journal of Obstetrics & Gynaecology. 2020;**127**:e70-e112. DOI: 10.1111/1471-0528.16092

[15] Sildver K, Veerus P, Gissler M, Lang K, Pisarev H. Caesarean section

and operative vaginal delivery in Estonia and Finland from 1992 to 2016: Registry-based study. European Journal of Public Health. 2024;**34**(6):1205-1209

[16] Europeristat. European Perinatal Health Report. [place unknown] Europeristat. 2022:1-134. Available from: https://www.europeristat.com/wp-content/uploads/2022/11/Euro-Peristat_Fact_sheets_2022_for_upload.pdf

[17] Merriam AA, Ananth CV, Wright JD, Siddiq Z, D'Alton ME, Friedman AM. Trends in operative vaginal delivery, 2005-2013: A population-based study. BJOG: An International Journal of Obstetrics & Gynaecology. 2017;**124**:1365-1372. DOI: 10.1111/1471-0528.14553

[18] Dutywa A, Olorunfemi G, Mbodi L. Trends and determinants of operative vaginal delivery at two academic hospitals in Johannesburg, South Africa 2005-2019. International Journal of Environmental Research and Public Health. 2022;**19**:16182. DOI: 10.3390/ijerph192316182

[19] Mebratu A, Ahmed A, Zemeskel AG, Alemu A, Temesgen T, Molla W, et al. Prevalence, indications and fetal outcomes of operative vaginal delivery in sub-Saharan Africa, systematic review, and meta-analysis. BMC Women's Health. 2023;**23**:95. DOI: 10.1186/s12905-023-02224-3

[20] Wani R, Champawat C. A review on the role of instrumental delivery in modern obstetrics. Review Article the Indian Practitioner. 2019;**72**:30-33

[21] Martin WL, Hutchon SP. Mechanism and management of normal labour. Current Obstetrics and Gynaecology. 2004;**14**:301-308. DOI: 10.1016/j.curobgyn.2004.06.001

[22] Dutta A. Presentation and mechanism of labour. In: Chandraharan E, editor. Labour and Delivery. Vol. 11. Sapiens Publishing, LTD; 2021. pp. 1-7. DOI: 10.3843/glowm.414323

[23] Mottet N, Hotton E, Eckman-Lacroix A, Bourtembourg A, Metz JP, Cot S, et al. Safety and efficacy of the OdonAssist inflatable device for assisted vaginal birth: The BESANCON ASSIST study. American Journal of Obstetrics and Gynecology. 2024;**230**:S947-S958. DOI: 10.1016/j.ajog.2023.05.016

[24] Siggelkow W. Comparison of obstetrics efficacy and safety of the kiwi OmniCup with conventional vacuum extraction. Geburtsh Frauenheilk. 2014;**74**:146-151

[25] Andrewartha KWC. The evaluation of the obstetric vacuum extractor. In: Griffiths PSJWL, editor. Summer. Vol. 17. Australia: O and G Magazine, Highway Press; 2015. pp. 71-73

[26] Wong MS. Forceps delivery: Contemporary tips for a classic obstetrics tool. Contemporary OB/GYN. 2019;**64**:14-17

[27] Vacca A. Operative vaginal delivery: Clinical appraisal of a new vacuum extraction device. Australian and New Zealand Journal of Obstetrics and Gynaecology. 2001;**41**:156-160

[28] Skehan M. Simplifying the use of the kiwi vacuum. International Journal of Gynecology & Obstetrics. 2024;**166**:551-558. DOI: 10.1002/ijgo.15295

[29] Vacca A. Vacuum-assisted delivery, improving patient outcomes and protecting yourself from litigation. Suppl OBG Manag. 2004:S1-S12

[30] Laborie Medical Technology Corp. Kiwi Complete Vacuum Delivery System.

USA: Laborie Medical Technology Corp; 2024. pp. 1-1. Available from: https://www.laborie.com/product/kiwi/ [Accessed: December 21, 2024]

[31] Esakoff T, Cheng Y, Snowden J, Caughey A. Is operative vaginal delivery safe in the preterm fetus? American Journal of Obstetrics and Gynecology. 2013;**208**:S343

[32] Bligard KH, Lipsey KL, Young OM. Simulation training for operative vaginal delivery among obstetrics and gynaecology residents: A systematic review. Obstetrics and Gynecology. 2019;**134**(Suppl 1):16S-21S. DOI: 10.1097/AOG.0000000000003431

[33] Feeley C, Crossland N, Betran AP, Weeks A, Downe S, Kingdon C. Training and expertise in undertaking assisted vaginal delivery (AVD): A mixed methods systematic review of practitioner's views and experiences. Reproductive Health. 2021;**18**:92. DOI: 10.1186/s12978-021-01146-3

[34] World Health Organisation. Research Gaps and Needs to Optimize the Use of Assisted Vaginal Birth: Technical Brief. Geneva Switzerland: World Health Organisation; 2023

[35] Usman S, Hanidu A, Kovalenko M, Hassan WA, Lees C. The sonopartogram. American Journal of Obstetrics and Gynecology. 2023;**228**:S997-S1016. DOI: 10.1016/j.ajog.2022.06.027

[36] Ghi T, Dall'asta A. Sonographic evaluation of the fetal head position and attitude during labour. American Journal of Obstetrics and Gynecology. 2024;**230**:S890-S900. DOI: 10.1016/j.ajog.2022.06.003

[37] Malani SN, Shrivastava D, Raka MS. A comprehensive review of the role of artificial intelligence in obstetrics and gynecology. Cureus. 2023;**15**(2):e34891. DOI: 10.7759/cureus.34891

[38] Michalitsi K, Metallinou D, Diamanti A, Georgakopoulou VE, Kagkouras I, Tsoukala E, et al. Artificial intelligence in predicting the mode of delivery: A systematic review. Cureus. 2024;**16**(9):e69115. DOI: 10.7759/cureus.69115

[39] Staat B, Combs CA. SMFM special statement: Operative vaginal delivery: Checklists for performance and documentation. American Journal of Obstetrics and Gynecology. 2020;**222**:B15-B21. DOI: 10.1016/j.ajog.2020.02.011

[40] Rather H, Muglu J, Veluthar L, Sivanesan K. The art of performing a safe forceps delivery: A skill to revitalise. European Journal of Obstetrics and Gynecology and Reproductive Biology. 2016;**199**:49-54. DOI: 10.1016/j.ejogrb.2016.01.045

[41] Vacca A. Handbook of Vacuum Delivery in Obstetric Practice. 3rd ed. Brisbane, Australia: Vacca Research; 2009

[42] Vacca A. Reducing the risks of a vacuum delivery. Fetal and Maternal Medicine Review. 2006;**17**:301-315

[43] McQuivey RW. Vacuum-assisted delivery: A review. Journal of Maternal-Fetal and Neonatal Medicine. 2004;**16**:171-180. DOI: 10.1080/1476-7050400001706

[44] Ekéus C, Högberg U, Norman M. Vacuum-assisted birth and risk for cerebral complications in term newborn infants: A population-based cohort study. BMC Pregnancy and Childbirth. 2014;**14**:36

[45] Åberg K, Norman M, Pettersson K, Järnbert-Pettersson H, Ekéus C. Protracted

vacuum extraction and neonatal intracranial haemorrhage among infants born at term: A nationwide case-control study. Acta Obstetricia et Gynecologica Scandinavica. 2019;**98**:523-532. DOI: 10.1111/aogs.13519

[46] Towner D, Castro MA, Eby-Wilkens E, Gilbert WM. Effect of mode of delivery in nulliparous women on neonatal intracranial injury. The New England Journal of Medicine. 1999;**34**:1709-1714

[47] Menticoglou SM, Perlman M, Manning FA. High cervical spinal cord injury in neonates delivered with forceps: Report of 15 cases. Obstetrics and Gynecology. 1995;**86**:589-594

[48] Cornthwaite KR, Bahl R, Lattey K, Draycott T. Management of impacted fetal head at cesarean delivery. American Journal of Obstetrics and Gynecology. 2024;**230**:S980-S987. DOI: 10.1016/j.ajog.2022.10.037

[49] Cornthwaite K, Bahl R, Winter C, Wright A, Kingdom J, Walker KF, et al. Management of impacted fetal head at caesarean birth: Scientific impact paper No. 73 (June 2023). BJOG: An International Journal of Obstetrics & Gynaecology. 2023;**130**:e40-e64. DOI: 10.1111/1471-0528.17534

Chapter 9

Operative Vaginal Delivery: A Review and Public Health Perspectives

Efuetnkeng Bechem

Abstract

Instrumental delivery, also called assisted vaginal birth, is a procedure whereas vaginal delivery is accomplished with the use of instruments, namely forceps and vacuum extractors. This is an obstetrical procedure introduced since the Greek and Roman era (between 500 BC and 500 AD) but still remain a current practice today as WHO qualifies it to be one of the six critical function of basic emergency obstetric care. It is, therefore, a vital procedure to improve obstetrical care in resource-limited settings. The indications for an assisted vaginal birth can not only be maternal, foetal or both but it also depends on the technical capacity of the birth attendant as it is not void of complications. There has been a decline in the procedure that has been reported worldwide. Lack of adequate training, education of stakeholders and appropriate communication for behavioural change have been several factors identified as major setbacks affecting the use of AVB. Identifying these setbacks and exposing the advantages of this delivery method whilst enhancing on behavioural changes constitute public health perspectives in operative vaginal delivery.

Keywords: forceps, vacuum extraction, vaginal birth, caesarean section, behavioural change

1. Introduction

Assisted vaginal birth (also called instrumental delivery) is carried out to accomplish birth for the benefit of mothers and babies, but it is sometimes associated with significant morbidity for both. According to Verma, Spalding and Wilkinson et al., assisted vaginal birth (AVB), is referred to the act of carrying out a vaginal birth with the help of an instrument, such as a forceps or vacuum extractor [1]. It is also known as instrumental delivery or operative vaginal birth.

These two instruments are safe and reliable for assisted delivery of a child, but emphasis should be laid on appropriate indications and contraindications of the procedures. The benefits and risks to both the mother and her foetus of using either instrument or the dangers of alternative caesarean section delivery must be considered in each case. The choice of instrument should be made by considering the clinical circumstances, the skill of the health care provider and the acceptance of the woman. This procedure should be carried out by a trained and experienced healthcare provider with good judgmental ability with the instrument chosen.

The World Health Organisation (WHO) has indicated AVB to be one of the seven essential services in basic emergency obstetric care [2].

In the United States, assisted vaginal delivery represented 3.1% of all deliveries, according to national data in 2015 [3]. Forceps-assisted births accounted for 0.5% of vaginal births; vacuum-assisted births accounted for 2.6% of vaginal births and 83%of all instrument-AVBs [4]. There is a reported decline from 9% in 1990. For these two methods, the vacuum is disproportionately selected, with a vacuum-to-forceps delivery ratio approximating 4:1. However, the prevalence of assisted vaginal birth varies across geographic regions in the United States and even within states, suggesting an inadequate and random application of evidence-based guidelines for AVB, or even more, the decline expertise with the technique in some areas [4]. In the United States, the highest rates for both forceps and vacuum-assisted births are recorded in the Midwest, whilst the lowest forceps-assisted delivery rates were recorded in the Northeast and the lowest vacuum-assisted delivery rates in the South [4]. In a systematic review and meta-analysis in 2023 among 17 studies in sub-Saharan Africa, Mebratu et al. identified a pooled prevalence of operative vaginal delivery of 7.98% of all vaginal births [5].

The most frequent indications for AVB include foetal distress in the second stage of labour with an advanced station of the foetal head, a prolonged second stage of labour and maternal exhaustion during the second stage of labour. Knowing the risks associated with caesarean sections carried out during the second stage of labour compared to pre-labour or early labour caesarean sections, AVB can be a tool to reduce maternal and perinatal morbidity and mortality in the second stage of labour [6]. This is particularly important in resource-limited settings where women and their babies have reduced access to high-quality (i.e. effective, safe, efficient, equitable, timely and people-centred) care [7].

It has been noted a global trend in the decrease in the use of instrumental deliveries contrasts with the increased use of caesarean section in the last decades, most particularly in low- and middle-income countries (LMICs) [7]. Whilst AVB is inexistent in some LMICs, it has been observed that its use is currently more common in high-income countries than in LMICs [8]. It is thought that potential factors associated with the underuse of AVB may be such as lack of staff adequately trained to indicate and perform ABV, lack of functioning equipment, inadequate support and supervision for trained healthcare workers to perform AVB, fear of complications or blame in case of adverse outcomes, and concerns on maternal and foetal safety [9].

2. History of assisted vaginal birth

AVB has been described as far back as the sixth century BC in Hindu medicine. Other references are found during the Greco-Roman era in the writings of Hippocrates between 500 BC and 500 AD [10]. However, in this era, labour may have occurred for several days resulting in intrapartum foetal death. In these circumstances, the intervention consisted of the use of surgical instruments or even kitchen utensils with the sole purpose of extracting the dead foetus and preventing maternal mortality [11]. The invention of assisted vaginal delivery as a method of preventing both maternal and neonatal morbidity has developed over several centuries and has been kept guarded secretly over several years by its inventors.

The French-born surgeon Peter Chamberlen (c.1560–1631) has been attributed to the invention of the obstetric forceps in the seventeenth century. Chamberlens instrument was first used in 1735 Scotland and England in 1735, whilst, William Smellie (1697–1763), a famous British obstetrician, is described to have pioneered the evolution and the use of the forceps in England [11]. Smellie added a lock and the fenestrated blades to the forceps originally designed by Chamberlen. Other designs with longer and pelvic curved blades based on scientific study of pelvic measurements were invented. This resulted in better use of the forceps and reduced foetal trauma.

It was in 1849 that Dr. James Young, an English surgeon, first described vacuum extractors [12]. However, it was in the 1950s, that the Swedish obstetrician, Dr. Tage Malmström published a series of studies on vacuum extraction, that it became popular. By 1992, the number of forceps-assisted deliveries was outnumbered by the number of vacuum-assisted deliveries in the US, and it was estimated by 2000 that 66% of operative vaginal deliveries were vacuum-assisted deliveries [13].

3. Different types of instruments

There are two different instruments used in AVB. The obstetric forceps and the vacuum extractor.

3.1 The obstetric forceps

The obstetric forceps is a metallic instrument made to adapt on the foetal head, whilst the operator exerts a pull to expel the baby from the birth canal [14]. The forceps consist of a blade that is linked to a handle by a shank (**Figures 1** and **2**).

The blade is the part that fits the foetal head and has two curves: the cephalic curve to encompass and protect the foetal head and a pelvic curve to accommodate the

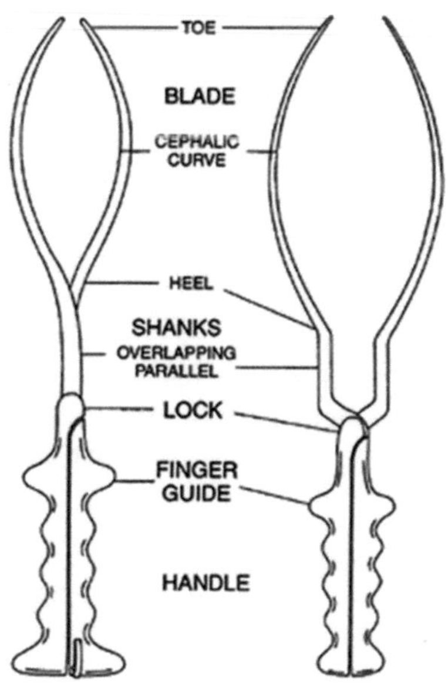

Figure 1.
Diagrammatic frontal view of an obstetrical forceps. Source [14].

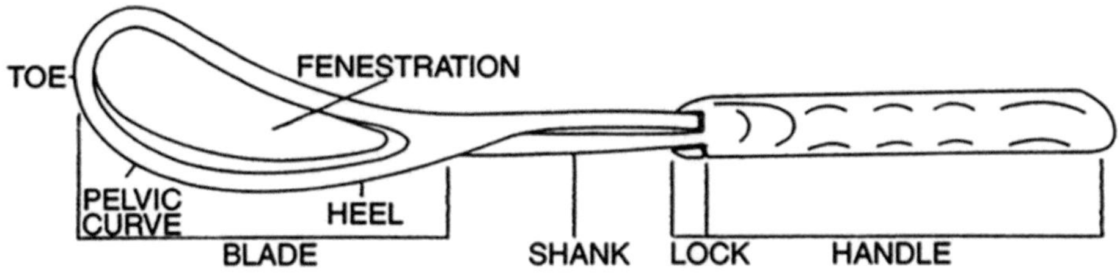

Figure 2.
Diagrammatic transverse view of an obstetrical forceps. Source [14].

maternal pelvic curve. It may be fenestrated or solid. The back of the blade is called the heel, whilst the tip is called the toe. The shanks may be parallel (Simpson-type forceps) or overlapping (Elliot-type forceps). The shank connects the blade to the handle *via* a lock (**Figure 1**). Several lock configurations exist, but the most common are the English and sliding locks. The handle is used for gripping the forceps by the operator to exert a pull force.

These features of the forceps were each designed for a purpose and the user needs to know before applying the forceps. Fenestrated blades prevent slippage on the baby's face by allowing the foetus's cheeks to bulge through, but they tend to leave bruise marks more easily than solid blades. Overlapping shanks provide more space towards the heel of the blades. This makes it preferable for the delivery of an infant with an unmolded head. The overlapping shanks also cause less stretching of the maternal perineum and, therefore, are better choices if rotation is attempted.

Several hundreds of different types of forceps exist, with the most commonly used being [15].

The Simpson forceps have a particular elongated cephalic curve. It is used when the head is impacted in the birth canal.

The Elliot forceps are designed with a rounded cephalic curve.

Kielland forceps have a shallow pelvic curve with a sliding lock. They are commonly used in rotatory delivery.

Wrigley's forceps are characterised by short shanks and blades to reduce the risk of maternal complications. It is most often used in deliveries in outlet forceps deliveries and caesarean deliveries.

Piper's forceps have downward-curving shanks to fit around the underside of the body of the foetus. It is typically used in the delivery of the after-coming head in breech presentation.

The criteria and technique for forceps deliveries are:

- Outlet forceps: The foetal skull is at the pelvic floor, and the scalp is visible at the introitus without separating labia. The sagittal suture in anterior-posterior diameter is in LOA, ROA or OA position. Rotation should be less than 45 degrees and the perineum crowns the foetal head.

- Low forceps: The foetal skull should be below +2 station, but not visible at the introitus. The rotation is less than 45 degrees in LOA or ROA to OA, and also in LOP or ROP to OP. Otherwise, rotation can be above 45 degrees.

- Mid forceps is when the station is above +2 and the head is engaged.

- High forceps have been abandoned.

3.2 Vacuum extraction

With the discovery of the vacuum extractor in 1849 by James Young, it was Malmström who developed a prototype of a modern vacuum extractor. His prototype is a metal cup and a flat plate it attached to a chain [16]. The chain is then placed in a rubber tube that helps to develop the vacuum and attached to a traction bar. Upon pulling, traction is applied to the cup by the chain and plate.

The silastic cup has replaced the metal cup in most devices. It has many advantages over the metal cup, most especially the rapid development of the vacuum and, therefore, pressure can be released between contractions, which decreases injury to the foetal head due to abrasions.

The metal-cup vacuum extractor has a mushroom-shaped cup in metal with a diameter varying from 40 to 60 mm. It is centrally attached to a chain connecting the cup to a detachable handle, used to apply traction. The metal cup is attached to a suction pump (mechanical or electrical suction device) *via* a peripheral vacuum.

The metal cup has the advantage of higher success rates and ease of use in the occiput-posterior position. However, the non-flexibility of metal cups makes their application on the foetal head difficult and uncomfortable and, therefore, associated with increased risk of foetal scalp injuries.

Soft-cup devices are usually used with a manual or an electrical suction device. Some are manufactured with a built-in vacuum-release valve that allows a controlled and rapidly attained pressure. This makes the manipulation easier and simpler for the operator. Soft-cup vacuum extractors are disposable or reusable.

Contrary to metal-cup devices, soft-cup vacuum devices cause lesser neonatal scalp injuries but with a higher failure rate.

Soft-cup vacuum extractors are usually bell or funnel-shaped. Some varieties, such as the mushroom-shaped vacuum cup, have the combined advantages of both metal and soft cups. Its soft sidewall reduces infant scalp trauma compared to the traditional Malmström metal cup.

3.3 Comparative advantages of forceps and vacuum extractors

- Forceps

Reduced neonatal injuries, such as retinal haemorrhage, cephalohematoma and transient lateral rectus palsy.

Higher successful rates of vaginal births

- Vacuum extractors

Quicker foetal delivery.
Easier to learn.
Lesser maternal discomfort.

Lesser maternal genital trauma.
Fewer neonatal craniofacial injuries.
Less anaesthesia required.

4. Indications of instrumental deliveries

Assisted vaginal delivery is generally performed to shorten the second phase of labour during delivery if the foetal heart tones are not reassuring or there is maternal exhaustion. Also, AVB is usually used to shorten the second phase of labour in cases when the mother has chronic medical conditions, such as heart disease, sickle cell disease or hypertension.

5. Prerequisite for assisted vaginal delivery

AVBs are at times called surgical vaginal deliveries because it entails a surgical procedure to deliver the baby vaginally. This means there should be appropriate training of the practitioner on the procedure, acquired experience and a robust indication. Complications usually occur when some conditions are not met before the procedure. According to Chawanpaiboon et al., 18.8% of maternal complications were recorded in all AVBs in a series in the US [17]. These conditions vary as per the method chosen.

5.1 Prerequisite for forceps delivery

For a successful forceps delivery, the examiner should be assured of a fully dilated cervix, an empty bladder and an engaged head presentation. The exact position of the head is also important to identify possible rotatory movements.

It is also primordial to know the type of the pelvis as only an adequate pelvis may accommodate an instrument.

The operator should know the different types of forceps available and be familiar with them.

Being an operative procedure, a forceps delivery should respect all the necessary aseptic measures for surgery and anaesthesia [14].

5.2 Prerequisite for vacuum extraction

Similar conditions are required to perform a vacuum extraction for vaginal birth.

A fully dilated cervix with an empty maternal bladder, the foetal head should be engaged membranes ruptured an adequate pelvis and appropriate anaesthesia and the respect of aseptic surgical measures.

Contrary to some forceps delivery done for the after-coming head in breech presentation, vacuum extraction is exclusively used in cephalic presentation.

In all AVB, a backup setting for caesarean delivery should be readily available in case of failure of the instrumental vaginal birth.

6. Complications of AVB

6.1 Maternal complications

Several maternal complications reported have contributed tremendously to the reduction in the use of instrumental deliveries [4]. Maternal complications may include:

- Post-partum haemorrhage
- Birth canal injury
- Uterine rupture
- Obstetrical fistula
- Urinary incontinence.

6.2 Neonatal complications

Complications to the new-born may include [18].

- Skull fracture
- Brain damage
- Cerebral palsy
- Cephalohaematoma
- Erb's syndrome

7. Contraindication of AVB

These are conditions that do not comply with the prerequisite outlined above. These include:

- An unengaged head
- An unknown foetal position
- Incomplete cervical dilatation
- Vacuum extraction is contra-indicated in pregnancy terms below 34 weeks for risk of intracranial haemorrhage.

8. Public health perspectives of assisted vaginal deliver

8.1 Challenges on the use of AVB

With assisted vaginal birth representing about 3.1% of all deliveries in the US [3], whilst about 7.98% in sub-Saharan Africa [5], there is a major disparity in the prevalence. This may explain why AVB prevalence is income and society related.

The decline in the use of assisted vaginal delivery over the years is quite noticeable [4].

The World Health Organisation has identified the lack of trained and experienced providers with abilities to identify women in labour that could benefit from AVB and also perform the procedure safely, as a major setback for its use. Training of providers is, therefore, considered a crucial aspect of capacity building in conducting AVB and as Feeley et al. reported, it would be welcomed by healthcare providers [19]. Meanwhile, it is a complex task to acquire and maintain AVB skills, which necessitate a supportive environment, supervision, mentorship and accountability.

On-site training and hands-on technique sessions are necessary to ensure the safe and sustainable use of instrumental deliveries.

In its intrapartum care for positive childbirth experience recommendations, the WHO recognises a 'positive childbirth experience' as a major pregnancy endpoint for all women and babies [20]. In this perspective, not only what is done that matters but also why, when and how it is done. It is, therefore, important for caregivers to develop non-clinical skills, such as effective information, education and communication skills, appropriate attitude in a multidisciplinary professional team, shared and consensual decision-making and how to build positive relationships among the pregnant woman, her family and the community.

Some cultural factors and challenges, such as poor understanding about the safety and benefits of an instrumental delivery compared to caesarean delivery in the second stage of labour, are to be addressed by stakeholders (e.g., pregnant women, families, obstetricians, midwives, anesthesiologists, neonatologists and healthcare managers). In many LMICs where there is a lack of trained medical doctors, regulations for the practice of AVB by midwives are not available and may expose them to professional litigations.

The absence of contextual guidelines on indications, contraindications procedural measures for AVB and decisions to follow after a failed attempt, are also limiting the use of AVB.

8.2 The way forward

When adequately indicated and practised, high-quality assisted vaginal delivery has the potential to reduce maternal and neonatal morbidity and mortality whilst preserving the mother from caesarean delivery. Currently, overuse of caesarean sections in some settings coexists with a good proportion of women not accessing life-saving procedures. The good introduction of AVB, and its sustainability when and where appropriate, is a complex challenge that requires multi-sector interventions that involve all stakeholders. The cost-effectiveness of AVB compared to caesarean sections is a clear indication to advocate for its promotion in LMICs.

Multidisciplinary and comprehensive approaches are necesary to address these cultural behaviours and relationships among stakeholders. Care receivers' and givers' experiences, beliefs and values about AVB and an alternative caesarean delivery are crucial and need to be considered to improve and optimise the design and implementation of good strategies.

Research on this aspect should not only consider AVB as a sole aspect but also the physiology, management and health-economic aspects of AVB and its alternatives. This should be embedded in a complete process to reintroduce AVB as a measure to improve healthcare in the capacity of givers benefits and safety whilst evaluating the providers' skills and experience. Handing down ok knowledge to junior colleagues is also another aspect that should be emphasised by policymakers to sustain this practice. The identification and treatment of complications that arise will reassure stakeholders.

The recognition of AVB as a practice within health systems, whilst identifying local challenges, limitations and priorities should be researched. The use of behavioural operational implementation research on systems thinking approach and behavioural changes to adapt to local realities are encouraged to ascertain the cultural difficulties around AVB [21]. Behavioural studies have been used on community cultural changes to impact the implementation of medical procedures [22].

9. Conclusion

Assisted vaginal delivery is an obstetrical practice that has been used for ages and continues to play a vital role in the shortening of the second stage of labour for various indications. Despite this pivotal position in obstetric care, its use has been declining over the years and replaced by caesarean delivery.

The WHO defined AVB as one of the basic obstetrical care. However, this declining trend has been caused by several factors, especially personnel training. In LMICs where health accessibility is not optimal with mostly out-of-pocket payment of healthcare, assisted vaginal delivery should be rather promoted as it is cost-effective to the system.

In this chapter, we identified some public health challenges hindering the use of instruments in childbirth and outlined some way forward. This is basically around the training of operators who should master the different instruments, have a robust indication, and avoid contraindications, clearly understand the per-requisite before using the instrument, and know practically how to use the devices; health education and communication of stakeholders involved, and finally advocacy for cultural change through behavioural approaches.

Conflict of interest

The authors declare no conflict of interest.

Author details

Efuetnkeng Bechem
Cite Des Palmiers District Hospital, Douala, Cameroon

*Address all correspondence to: befuetnkeng@yahoo.fr

References

[1] Verma GL, Spalding JJ, Wilkinson MD, Hofmeyr GJ, Vannevel V, O'Mahony F. Instruments for assisted vaginal birth. Cochrane Database of Systematic Reviews. 2021;**2021**:CD005455. DOI: 10.1002/14651858.CD005455.pub3

[2] World Health Organization, United Nations Population Fund, Mailman School of Public Health. Averting Maternal Death and Disability & United Nations Children's Fund (UNICEF). Monitoring Emergency Obstetric Care: A Handbook. Geneva: World Health Organization; 2009. Available from: https://iris.who.int/handle/10665/44121

[3] Cunningham F, Leveno KJ, Dashe JS, Hoffman BL, Spong CY, Casey BM, editors. Operative vaginal delivery. In: Williams Obstetrics, 26e. New York: McGraw Hill; 2022. Available from: https://obgyn.mhmedical.com/content.aspx?bookid=2977&sectionid=252979298 [Accessed: August 06, 2024]

[4] Clark SL, Belfort MA, Hankins GD, Meyers JA, Houser FM. Variation in the rates of operative delivery in the United States. American Journal of Obstetrics and Gynecology. 2007;**196**(6):526.e1-526.e5. DOI: 10.1016/j.ajog.2007.01.024

[5] Mebratu A, Ahmed A, Zemeskel AG, Alemu A, Temesgen T, Molla W, et al. Prevalence, indications and fetal outcomes of operative vaginal delivery in sub-Saharan Africa, systematic review, and meta-analysis. BMC Women's Health. 2023;**23**(1):95. DOI: 10.1186/s12905-023-02224-3

[6] Pattinson RC, Vannevel V, Barnard D, Baloyi S, Gebhardt GS, Le Roux K, et al. Failure to perform assisted deliveries is resulting in an increased neonatal and maternal morbidity and mortality: An expert opinion. South African Medical Journal. 2018;**108**(2):75-78. DOI: 10.7196/SAMJ.2017.v108i2.12786

[7] Sobhy S, Arroyo-Manzano D, Murugesu N, Karthikeyan G, Kumar V, Kaur I, et al. Maternal and perinatal mortality and complications associated with caesarean section in low-income and middle-income countries: A systematic review and meta-analysis. Lancet. 2019;**393**(10184):1973-1982. DOI: 10.1016/S0140-6736(18)32386-9. Epub 2019 Mar 28

[8] Bailey PE. The disappearing art of instrumental delivery: Time to reverse the trend. International Journal of Gynaecology and Obstetrics. 2005;**91**(1):89-96. DOI: 10.1016/j.ijgo.2005.05.016

[9] Crossland N, Kingdon C, Balaam MC, Betran AP, Downe S. Women's, partners' and healthcare providers' views and experiences of assisted vaginal birth: A systematic mixed methods review. Reproductive Health. 2020;**17**(1):83. DOI: 10.1186/s12978-020-00915-w

[10] Low JA. Operative delivery: Yesterday and today. Journal of Obstetrics and Gynaecology Canada. 2009;**31**(2):132-141. DOI: 10.1016/s1701-2163(16)34097-x

[11] Sheikh S, Ganesaratnam I, Jan H. The birth of forceps. JRSM Short Reports. 2013;**4**(7):1-4. DOI: 10.1177/2042533313478412

[12] Ali UA, Norwitz ER. Vacuum-assisted vaginal delivery. Reviews in Obstetrics and Gynecology. 2009 Winter;**2**(1):5-17

[13] Attilakos G, Sibanda T, Winter C, et al. A randomised controlled trial of

a new handheld vacuum extraction device. BJOG: An International Journal of Obstetrics and Gynaecology. 2005;**112**:1510-1515

[14] Charles A. Gynecologic care of HIV-infected women. The Global Library of Women's Medicine. 2011;**10**:31. DOI: 10.3843/GLOWM.1013. ISSN: 1756-2228

[15] Patel RR, Murphy DJ. Forceps delivery in modern obstetric practice. BMJ. 2004;**328**(7451):1302-1305. DOI: 10.1136/bmj.328.7451.1302

[16] Jeon J, Na S. Vacuum extraction vaginal delivery: Current trend and safety. Obstetrics & Gynecology Science. 2017;**60**(6):499-505. DOI: 10.5468/ogs.2017.60.6.499. Epub 2017 Oct 23

[17] Chawanpaiboon S, Titapant V, Pooliam J. Maternal complications and risk factors associated with assisted vaginal delivery. BMC Pregnancy and Childbirth. 2023;**23**(1):756. DOI: 10.1186/s12884-023-06080-9

[18] Chawanpaiboon S, Titapant V, Pooliam J. Neonatal complications and risk factors associated with assisted vaginal delivery. Scientific Reports. 2024;**14**:11960. DOI: 10.1038/s41598-024-62703-x

[19] Feeley C, Crossland N, Betran AP, Weeks A, Downe S, Kingdon C. Training and expertise in undertaking assisted vaginal delivery (AVD): A mixed methods systematic review of practitioners' views and experiences. Reproductive Health. 2021;**18**(1):92. DOI: 10.1186/s12978-021-01146-3

[20] World Health Organization. WHO Recommendations: Intrapartum Care for a Positive Childbirth Experience. Geneva, Switzerland: World Health Organization; 2018. Available from: https://iris.who.int/handle/10665/260178 [Assessed: August 15, 2024]

[21] Adam T, de Savigny D. Systems thinking for strengthening health systems in LMICs: Need for a paradigm shift. Health Policy and Planning. 2012;**27 Suppl 4**:iv1-iv3. DOI: 10.1093/heapol/czs084

[22] Ghebreyesus TA. Using behavioural science for better health. Bulletin of the World Health Organization. 2021;**99**(11):755. DOI: 10.2471/BLT.21.287387

Chapter 10

Cost-Benefit and Outcome Comparison: Operative Vaginal and Cesarean Delivery

Habtamu Alemu Tena and Tesfahun Simon Hadaro

Abstract

Operative vaginal delivery (OVD) is a critical obstetric intervention that significantly reduces maternal and neonatal morbidity and mortality. This study, drawing from recent literature, provides a comprehensive overview of operative vaginal delivery (OVD), including its indications, contraindications, prerequisites, rate of OVD per region, and a cost-benefit analysis of comparing OVD to cesarean delivery (C-section), along with their respective healthcare outcomes. The finding of this study indicates that the rate of OVD has decreased over the past few decades, contributing to the increase in cesarean delivery rates worldwide. Factors influencing the use of OVD include the availability of trained healthcare providers, cultural attitudes toward childbirth, healthcare infrastructure, and regional policies. In terms of healthcare cost, OVD is generally more cost-effective than C-sections, particularly in low-risk pregnancies, contributing to better maternal outcomes and lower healthcare costs. The study underscores the importance of a balanced approach to labor management, carefully weighing the benefits and risks of OVD against the rising trend of C-sections. The findings have significant implications for healthcare policy and clinical practice aimed at improving maternal and neonatal health outcomes globally.

Keywords: operative delivery, operative vaginal delivery, instrumental delivery, cesarean delivery, spontaneous vaginal delivery, healthcare outcomes

1. Introduction

Operative vaginal delivery (OVD) involves using specialized obstetric instruments, such as forceps or vacuum devices, to assist in the vaginal delivery of a fetus, particularly when the natural progression of labor is hindered, posing risks to both mother and infant. This intervention is recommended to expedite the second stage of labor and reduce the need for second-stage cesarean deliveries, lowering associated morbidity and mortality [1]. Its importance is especially pronounced in low- and middle-income countries, where a shortage of skilled healthcare providers and limited access to necessary equipment restricts its widespread use [2].

Despite its proven efficacy, the utilization and perception of OVD have varied widely across different regions and healthcare systems, influenced by factors such as clinical expertise, training availability, and cultural attitudes toward childbirth [3].

IntechOpen

From a public health perspective, understanding the implications of OVD is crucial. Careful consideration of the balance between its benefits and potential risks is essential to inform guidelines and policies that optimize maternal and neonatal outcomes [3, 4].

Recent trends indicate a decline in OVD rates in favor of rising C-section rates, sparking debates about the best practices for managing labor and delivery. This shift raises concerns about the long-term health implications for mothers and infants, as well as the economic burden on healthcare systems [5, 6]. Operative vaginal delivery is used to achieve or expedite safe vaginal delivery for maternal or fetal indications, such as prolonged second stage of labor, non-reassuring fetal heart rate patterns in the second stage of labor, maternal exhaustion, and an inability to push effectively; medical indications such as maternal cardiac disease and a need to avoid pushing in the second stage of labor [7, 8].

Contraindications to operative vaginal delivery (OVD) include both maternal and fetal factors that increase the risk of complications. These include pelvic abnormalities, incomplete cervical dilatation, inadequate maternal effort, active genital infections, unengaged fetal head, fetal malpresentation (such as breech or face presentation), fetal bleeding disorders, and suspected macrosomia. Proper assessment of these factors is crucial to minimize risks and ensure a safe delivery for both mother and baby [9–11].

The prerequisites for operative vaginal delivery (OVD) include informed consent from the mother, a fully dilated cervix, an engaged fetal head, adequate anesthesia, ruptured membranes, and an adequate pelvis. Additionally, there must be readiness for a potential cesarean delivery if necessary, and there should be no contraindications such as cephalopelvic disproportion or fetal bleeding disorders. Meeting these criteria is essential to ensure a safe and successful OVD and to achieve favorable outcomes [12–14].

Operative vaginal delivery (OVD) can lead to successful vaginal deliveries, reducing the need for cesarean sections. However, it also poses significant risks to the mother and the baby. Both maternal and fetal complications can arise from OVD, making skilled technique and careful clinical decision-making essential. Maternal complications can include perineal tears, hemorrhage, pelvic floor dysfunction, infection, and urinary or fecal incontinence. For the fetus, potential risks range from scalp lacerations and cephalohematoma to more serious conditions like subgaleal hemorrhage, intracranial hemorrhage, or facial nerve palsy [15–17]. These risks highlight the importance of precise clinical execution, appropriate patient selection, and diligent monitoring during and after the procedure to minimize harm to the mother and the child.

When performed by experienced clinicians, with careful patient selection and proper technique, the outcomes of OVD can be favorable. The procedure often prevents the need for a cesarean section, which carries its own set of risks, including hemorrhage, infection, prolonged healing, and higher costs. Long-term morbidities are notable, such as the increased likelihood of repeat cesarean deliveries, complications during a trial of labor after cesarean (TOLAC), and placental abnormalities, including placenta accreta. Therefore, the decision to proceed with OVD must be carefully weighed against these potential risks, and close monitoring of both the mother and neonate is critical during and after the procedure to ensure favorable outcomes.

Several public health issues emerge when evaluating OVD. These include the accessibility and quality of obstetric care, the training and proficiency of healthcare providers in performing OVD, and the socioeconomic and demographic factors influencing the choice of delivery method [18]. Moreover, disparities in the availability and utilization of OVD highlight the need for equitable healthcare provision and the importance of addressing systemic barriers that prevent optimal care [17]. By reviewing existing literature, this study seeks to provide comprehensive insights into the benefits and challenges associated with OVD, ultimately contributing to more informed policy-making and improved healthcare outcomes.

2. Background statistics of OVD performed per region per year

Operative vaginal delivery (OVD) statistics vary across regions and years based on recent literature. These statistics highlight the variability in OVD rates across different regions, influenced by a combination of healthcare practices, the availability of trained professionals, and cultural factors.

The United Kingdom and France have the highest OVD rates, ranging from 10–15% [9, 19]. This is consistent with the broader trends observed in Europe, where OVD is a common practice due to better access to healthcare and skilled birth attendants.

The rate of operative vaginal delivery (OVD) in Africa varies significantly across different regions, with the lowest prevalence in sub-Saharan Africa, due to limited access to skilled birth attendants and necessary equipment. A systematic review and meta-analysis revealed an overall pooled prevalence of OVD at 7.98% across 17 studies involving 190,900 births, reflecting the challenges in the healthcare infrastructure. Specific indications for OVD included prolonged second stage of labor (32.81%) and non-reassuring fetal heart rate (37.35%) [20].

The rate of operative vaginal delivery (OVD) in the United States and Canada has been notably low compared to other countries. Recent studies indicate that the OVD rate in the U.S. is approximately 3.1%, with forceps being used in only 0.5% of deliveries. Both countries have seen a decline in OVD rates, now ranging from 3 to 5% [21, 22]. This decline is attributed to changes in obstetric practices and increased preference for cesarean sections in certain clinical scenarios.

Brazil and Argentina also have relatively low OVD rates, with Brazil having the lowest at around 1–3%. These countries have relatively low OVD rates. Brazil, in particular, has one of the lowest rates, ranging from 1–3%. This low rate is influenced by the high rates of cesarean sections, which are often preferred over OVD in these regions [23, 24].

The rate of operative vaginal delivery (OVD) in Asia varies significantly across different regions and healthcare settings. Research indicates that while OVD is an essential skill in obstetrics, its utilization remains low in many areas. In Singapore, the rate of OVD was approximately 10% from 2012 to 2017, with a balanced use of forceps and vacuum extractors. A study in Nepal reported a much lower frequency of 2.3% among 3060 deliveries, primarily used in nulliparous women, with fetal distress being the most common indication [25, 26].

The OVD rate in Australia and New Zealand is around 10–12%, with a preference for vacuum over forceps [18]. Asia: India: OVD rates in India vary significantly by region, ranging from 2 to 5% [27, 28]. Urban areas tend to have higher rates due to better access to healthcare facilities. China's OVD rates are relatively low, around 2.3%, as cesarean sections are more commonly preferred for complicated deliveries [29].

These findings highlight the significant regional differences in OVD practices, influenced by factors such as healthcare infrastructure, training of healthcare

Region	Country	OVD rates
Europe	United Kingdom	10–15%
	France	Comparable to the UK
	Germany	7–10%
Africa	Sub-Saharan Africa	7.98%
North America	United States	3–5%
	Canada	3–4%
Latin America	Brazil	1–3%
	Argentina	3–5%
Asia	India	2–5%
	China	2–5%
	Singapore	10%
	Nepal	2.3%
Australia and New Zealand	Australia	10–12%
	New Zealand	Comparable to Australia

Note: Data adapted from sources [9, 18–29] numbered as per sources used in the compilation of **Table 1**.

Table 1.
Operative vaginal delivery rates across regions and countries.

providers, and cultural preferences regarding childbirth methods. **Table 1** presents an overview of OVD statistics across different regions.

3. A cost-benefit analysis of OVD vs. cesarean delivery and comparative healthcare outcomes

The decision between operative vaginal delivery and cesarean delivery (CD) is crucial in obstetric care, with significant implications for healthcare costs and outcomes. Recent studies provide insights into the cost-benefit analysis of these delivery methods and their comparative healthcare outcomes. The analysis considers factors such as hospital costs and maternal and neonatal health outcomes. Cesarean sections, particularly in low-risk pregnancies, are linked to higher healthcare costs, poorer perinatal outcomes, and increased rates of maternal and neonatal complications, making them a lower-value delivery option [30].

Studies showed that OVD is generally more cost-effective and associated with better maternal outcomes compared to cesarean delivery (C-section), particularly in low-risk pregnancies. Successful OVD has been associated with a 45% reduction in severe maternal complications without increasing the risk of severe neonatal morbidity compared to cesarean delivery after a prolonged second stage of labor. This reduction in maternal morbidity also helps lower overall healthcare costs. Furthermore, OVD has been associated with shorter hospital stays, quicker recovery periods, lower infection rates, and higher rates of immediate breastfeeding initiation (92.57% for vaginal births compared to 88.43% for cesarean deliveries) [31, 32].

From a cost perspective, vaginal deliveries, including OVD, generally incur lower costs than C-sections due to shorter hospital stays, fewer surgical resources, and reduced postoperative care needs. Cesarean sections, on the other hand, have both higher direct and indirect costs. These include longer hospitalizations, increased medical supplies, and a higher incidence of neonatal intensive care unit (NICU) admissions for newborns (6.7% for cesareans vs. 4.5% for vaginal births). Furthermore, cesarean deliveries lead to more maternal ICU admissions (0.8 vs. 0.3% for vaginal births), which also drives up healthcare expenses [33, 34].

Long-term risks associated with cesarean deliveries include uterine rupture and placenta previa in future pregnancies. They also increase the likelihood of chronic health conditions, such as pelvic floor dysfunction or issues related to adhesions. OVD, when performed properly, avoids many of these risks and preserves the option to deliver vaginally in the future. Although both delivery methods can be life-saving when necessary, OVD provides better maternal outcomes and is generally more cost-effective, especially in low-risk situations. It also contributes to reducing the rates of primary cesarean deliveries and mitigating long-term maternal health complications [35, 36].

These findings emphasize the importance of carefully considering the mode of delivery to optimize maternal and neonatal outcomes while managing healthcare costs effectively. It is essential for informing healthcare policies aimed at optimizing delivery methods, balancing costs, and improving overall maternal and neonatal outcomes.

4. Conclusion

The finding of this study indicates that operative vaginal delivery (OVD) is a crucial intervention in obstetrics, significantly reducing maternal and neonatal morbidity and mortality while being more cost-effective than cesarean delivery, particularly in low-risk pregnancies. It highlights a concerning trend of declining OVD rates in favor of increasing cesarean sections, which are associated with higher complications and costs. The study emphasizes the need for equitable healthcare access to OVD and calls for informed policy-making to promote its use, ensuring that all women can benefit from safe and effective delivery methods. Overall, the findings advocate for a balanced approach to labor management that carefully weighs the benefits and risks of OVD against the rising preference for cesarean deliveries, ultimately aiming to improve maternal and neonatal health outcomes globally.

Conflict of interest

The authors declare no conflict of interest.

Author details

Habtamu Alemu Tena* and Tesfahun Simon Hadaro
Arba Minch University, Arba Minch, Ethiopia

*Address all correspondence to: habtishmid84@gmail.com

References

[1] Peaceman AM. Operative vaginal birth: ACOG practice bulletin, number 219. Obstetrics and Gynecology. 1 Apr 2020;**135**(4):E149-E159

[2] Daniel K, Daly R, Elizabeth T, Eimear W, Enya F, Roisin G, et al. 704 Operative vaginal delivery rates over two-decades: Instrument choice and neonatal morbidity- implications for resident training. American Journal of Obstetrics and Gynecology. 2024. DOI: 10.1016/j.ajog.2023.11.730

[3] Vannevel V, Swanepoel C, Pattinson RC. Global perspectives on operative vaginal deliveries. Best Practice and Research. Clinical Obstetrics and Gynaecology. 2019;**56**:107-113

[4] Miller HE, Danielle M. How are maternal and neonatal outcomes impacted by the contemporary practice of operative vaginal delivery? OBGM. 2022;**34**(4):49-50. Available from: https://www.mdedge.com/obgyn/article/253989/obstetrics/how-arematernal-and-neonatal-outcomesimpacted-contemporary

[5] Balla PC, Nallapu SSR. A review of caesarean section rates in India: Causes for increased prevalence and suggestions for a rational approach. International Journal of Reproduction, Contraception, Obstetrics and Gynecology. 2022;**11**(4):1324-1328

[6] Angolile CM, Max BL, Mushemba J, Mashauri HL. Global increased cesarean section rates and public health implications: A call to action. Health Science Reports. 2023;**6**(5):e1274

[7] Svelato A, Carabaneanu A, Sergiampietri C, Mannella P, D'Avino S, De Luca C, et al. "To get the baby out off the hook": A prospective, longitudinal, multicenter, observational study about decision making in vacuum-assisted operative vaginal delivery. BMC Pregnancy and Childbirth. 2022;**22**(1):128

[8] Skotalczyk M, Łokczewska-Bojar A, Kuziemkowska D, Łącka-Majcher A, Tarsa G, Kępka P, et al. Operative vaginal deliveries – A relic of the past or a promising prospect? Journal of Education, Health and Sport. 2023;**16**:226-241

[9] O'Brien S, ElHodaiby M, Draycott T. Operative vaginal birth. In: Jha S, Ferriman E, editors. Medicolegal Issues in Obstetrics and Gynaecology. Cham: Springer International Publishing; 2018. pp. 139-145. DOI: 10.1007/978-3-319-78683-4_26

[10] Aimakhu CO, Ilesanmi AO. Operative vaginal delivery. In: Okonofua F, Balogun JA, Odunsi K, Chilaka VN, editors. Contemporary Obstetrics and Gynecology for Developing Countries. Cham: Springer International Publishing; 2021. pp. 175-192. DOI: 10.1007/978-3-030-75385-6_16

[11] Masturzo B, Zonca M, Germano C, Girlando F, Diacono D, Attini R, et al. Operative vaginal delivery: All you should know. Minerva Obstetrics and Gynecology. 2021;**73**(1):45-56

[12] Horan MA, Murphy DJ. Operative vaginal delivery. Obstetrics, Gynaecology and Reproductive Medicine. 2016;**26**(12):358-363

[13] Oduola O, Garry N, Murphy DJ. Operative vaginal birth. Obstetrics, Gynaecology and Reproductive Medicine. 2020;**30**(1):19-25

[14] Yeomans ER. Operative vaginal delivery. Obstetrics and Gynecology. 2010;**115**(3):645-653

[15] Abbas RA, Qadi YH, Bukhari R, Shams T. Maternal and neonatal complications resulting from vacuum-assisted and normal vaginal deliveries. Cureus. May 2021;**13**(5)

[16] Nedamo SA, Sakelo AN, Tirore LL, Abate AA. Maternal complications related to operative vaginal delivery and their associated factors among women delivered at NEMCS hospital, Southwest Ethiopia. Obstetrics and Gynecology International. 2023;**2023**(1):4214252

[17] Deane RP. Operative vaginal delivery and pelvic floor complications. Best Practice and Research Clinical Obstetrics and Gynaecology. 1 Apr 2019;**56**:81-92

[18] TsakiridisI, GioulekaS, MamopoulosA, Athanasiadis A, Daniilidis A, Dagklis T. Operative vaginal delivery: A review of four national guidelines. Journal of Perinatal Medicine. 2020;**48**(3):189-198. DOI: 10.1515/jpm-2019-0433

[19] Sainz JA, Borrero C, García-Mejido JA. Forceps application with intrapartum ultrasonography. In: Intrapartum Ultrasonography for Labor Management. 2nd ed. Berlin: Springer; 2021. pp. 369-383

[20] Mebratu A, Ahmed A, Zemeskel AG, Alemu A, Temesgen T, Molla W, et al. Prevalence, indications and fetal outcomes of operative vaginal delivery in sub-Saharan Africa, systematic review, and meta-analysis. BMC Women's Health. 2023;**23**(1):95-97

[21] Okram S, Betha K, Bodhanapati J, Tejasri K. Forceps deliveries and fetomaternal outcome in modern obstetrics. International Journal of Reproduction, Contraception, Obstetrics and Gynecology. 2019;**8**:4862

[22] Dunk SA, Owen J, Lu MY, Kim DJ, Szychowski JM, Subramaniam A. Operative vaginal delivery as an independent risk factor for maternal postpartum infectious morbidity. American Journal of Obstetrics and Gynecology MFM. 2022;**4**(6):100705

[23] Prospective A. Population-based study of trends in operative vaginal delivery compared to Cesarean delivery rates in low- and middle-income countries, 2010-2016. American Journal of Perinatology. 2019;**36**(7):730-736

[24] Ghanchi FM, Mansuri MI, Doshi HU, PHK P. Maternal and perinatal outcome in instrumental vaginal deliveries over 5 years: A retrospective study. International Journal of Reproduction, Contraception, Obstetrics and Gynecology. 2023;**12**(4):934-939

[25] Joshi R, Shrestha S, Chaudhary J, Pandit U, Tamrakar R. Fetomaternal outcome in operative vaginal deliveries in a tertiary care centre: A descriptive retrospective study. Journal of BP Koirala Institute of Health Sciences. 2020;**3**(2):23-27

[26] Zhang VRY, Tan EL, Edison PE, Kanagalingam D. Operative vaginal delivery: Practice patterns and outcomes at a tertiary general hospital. Singapore Medical Journal. 2023;**64**(5):313-318

[27] Sultana MA, Suprada K, Bahadur BR, Rao KG. Instrumental deliveries and its outcome in tertiary care center. International Journal of Reproduction, Contraception, Obstetrics and Gynecology. 2024;**13**(6):1527-1530

[28] Al Riyami N, Al Salmiyah M, Khan D, Al RI. Maternal and neonatal outcomes of operative vaginal deliveries

at a single tertiary center. Oman Medical Journal. 2021;**36**(3):e263

[29] Wang X, Hellerstein S, Hou L, Zou L, Ruan Y, Zhang W. Caesarean deliveries in China. BMC Pregnancy and Childbirth. 2017;**17**(1):54

[30] Negrini R, da Silva Ferreira RD, Guimarães DZ. Value-based care in obstetrics: Comparison between vaginal birth and caesarean section. BMC Pregnancy and Childbirth. 2021;**21**(1):333

[31] Muraca GM, Boutin A, Razaz N, Lisonkova S, John S, Ting JY, et al. Maternal and neonatal trauma following operative vaginal delivery. CMAJ. 2022;**194**(1):E1-E12

[32] Phibbs CM, Kozhimannil KB, Leonard SA, Lorch SA, Main EK, Schmitt SK, et al. The effect of severe maternal morbidity on infant costs and lengths of stay. Journal of Perinatology. 2022;**42**(5):611-616

[33] Shah NT, Golen TH, Kim JG, Mistry B, Kaplan R, Gawande A. A cost analysis of hospitalization for vaginal and Cesarean deliveries [282]. Obstetrics and Gynecology. 2015;**125**:91S

[34] Mirparsa F, Mirzaei A, Alimohammadzadeh K. Cost analysis - The desirability of natural delivery and caesarean section with decision tree model. International Journal of Health Sciences: 47908-47921. Available from: https://sciencescholar.us/journal/index.php/ijhs/article/view/13402

[35] Panelli DM, Leonard SA, Judy A, El-Sayed YY, Gilbert W, Lyell DJ. 918: Sustaining the practice of operative vaginal delivery: Maternal and neonatal outcomes among a contemporary cohort. American Journal of Obstetrics and Gynecology. 2020;**222**(1):S568

[36] Ramphul M. "Strategies to increase the accuracy and safety of OVD" (clinical assessment skills and role of ultrasound, simulation training and new technologies to enhance instrument application). Best Practice and Research Clinical Obstetrics and Gynaecology. 2019;**56**:35-46